HOW I DEALT WITH
CANCER
IN A NON-CONVENTIONAL WAY

Gloria Austin

BALBOA.
PRESS

A DIVISION OF HAY HOUSE

Balboa Press books may be ordered through booksellers or by contacting:

Balboa Press
A Division of Hay House
1663 Liberty Drive
Bloomington, IN 47403
www.balboapress.com
1 (877) 407-4847

Print information available on the last page.

ISBN: 978-1-5043-6238-2 (sc)
ISBN: 978-1-5043-6260-3 (e)

Balboa Press rev. date: 07/18/2016

CONTENTS

DEDICATION

How I Dealt with Cancer in a Non-Conventional Way, is dedicated to all those courageous enough to want to deal with cancer in a non-conventional way and are brave enough to do so.

EPIGRAPH

My brothers and sisters, whenever you face trials of any kind, consider it nothing but joy, because you know that the testing of your faith produces endurance; and let endurance have its effect, so that you may be mature and complete, lacking in nothing.

(James 1: 2, NRSV)

FOREWORD

For some strange reason, perhaps one connected to culture or pride, many people are reluctant to discuss their illnesses – or their *dis-ease*, as Gloria Austin would say. I am so happy that Gloria has placed no such limitation on herself. She shares generously about her dis-ease, and most important, the non-conventional way that she used to deal with it. The result is her simple, yet thought-provoking book, entitled, *How I Dealt with Cancer in a Non-Conventional Way,* from which those who have similar diagnoses can derive not only comfort, but guidance, on how to approach their recovery.

Her easy-to-apply methods and solutions draw upon our traditional treatments in the Caribbean. These are combined with spiritual principles that we have repeated through the ages, without true thought for their meaning. Gloria repeatedly tells us how she applied many of these scripture verses, with faith, and indeed how they have worked to help her recover.

One of the biblical statements that Gloria has brought into focus is found in Psalm 139:14, KJV, "*I will praise thee; for I am fearfully and wonderfully made: marvellous are thy works, and that my soul knoweth right well*". She has virtually adopted this principle as her mantra. For me, one of the most moving and powerful chapters in her book is Chapter 3, "*My Wonderfully-Made Body*". If there is nothing else that a reader ought to take away from this book, it is how to get deeply into the scripture and extract the wisdoms that lie imbedded within the verses. So no more superficial repetitions.

What also strikes me in the book is Gloria's decision to draw deeply from her culture, her roots and her past to respond to the diagnosis of cancer. Firstly, I could not help but feel resentful, however, at the fact that the treatments and concoctions that were applied in the old days have now become the "*non-conventional way*" of dealing with dis-eases. Modern medicine has expelled those traditional treatments and has now become the *conventional* way. It should, of course, be the other way around.

Our people did not see the importance of documenting, preserving and *improving on* the traditional methods. Instead, those methods were discarded and our people now cling tenaciously to modern approaches, the origins – and effects - of which, we are ignorant. In fact, some of these conventional methods incorporate the very traditional medicines, that our people rejected. Aloes and coconut oil are cases in point.

Secondly, Gloria's approach proves that when people are at their most vulnerable, they go back to their origins and roots. No matter how far we roam or what modern ideas we embrace, when the chips are down, we believe deep in our hearts that going back to base will help us. Thirdly, I am impressed by the fact that Gloria Austin was willing to do the necessary research on the non-conventional ways, apply her research and most of all, to share it in this book. Thank you so much, Gloria.

In conclusion, I heartily recommend to all of us, what I regard as Gloria's most powerful declaration in the book ... her avoidance of saying, "*I have cancer*". The reason? "*I did not own it as it is not something that I wanted*". "*I disarmed it by saying I was diagnosed with cancer*". That was a very profound idea for me. Thus she instructs us not to give the dis-ease a name. Think of it as a "*malfunction of my body… which can be repaired.*" Isn't this a refreshing and reassuring idea?

This book is indeed recommended reading for all persons. Our health ought to be our abiding concern. How do we make sure that we make decisions that preserve and repair our bodies when they malfunction – as they inevitably will? On this question, Gloria Austin's book, *How I Dealt with Cancer in a Non-Conventional Way*, is a true roadmap for each of us.

Deborah Moore-Miggins
LL.B., L.EC., LL.M, Hubert Humphrey Fellow (1992)
Co-Founder of the Tobago Newspapers Ltd, Director of the Empowerment
Foundation of Tobago
Coordinator of the Annual Tobago Word Festival
Author of, *The Caribbean Proverbs that Raised Us* &
British 'Other Ranks' – John Miggins' World War II Experiences

FOREWORD

I am both Gloria's family physician and her former neighbor. We passed interesting plants and our gardens' produce back and forth over the fence that separated our homes. I am so pleased that she has written this book. There are gems of information among its pages. These pearls of wisdom will help you to take control of your own health and well-being whether you have been diagnosed with a serious illness or you just want to optimize and maintain your mental, physical, emotional and spiritual well-being.

I truly believe that if you read this book and adopt even some of the philosophy that is shared, you can improve your experience of life. Contained within Gloria's story are basic tenets for living a full and rewarding life. Gloria explains absolute truths in clear and understandable ways:

- Our bodies are experts at healing.
- What we eat and how much we move our bodies affects our health.

- Our thoughts and beliefs affect our biology, our immune system, our mood.
- A feeling of deep connection to the divine (whatever you perceive that to be), improves outcomes in many illnesses.
- Social connections, friends and family, are important to us all and affect our health and well-being.

These are some of the truths explored.

One of the most important pieces of advice that is shared is, when diagnosed with any illness, the following steps should be followed:

- Learn as much as you can about that disease, gather information from reputable sources and evaluate it.
- Consider the information in the context of your own life and priorities and then follow your inner guidance to decide what course of treatment is best for you.
- Only you know all aspects of your life, you know what you value most at any given point in time, and really...you live with the consequences of your choices.
- Have a good therapeutic relationship with your doctor, one in which you can be heard and supported in your decision making.

Each chapter ends with a summary, bullet points of what has been covered in that chapter. This is useful when you forget Gloria's suggestions for living well. Looking at these points provide us with a quick and easy reminder of where we should direct our focus.

So delve deeply into this book, take your time to absorb it, read and re-read the chapters that inspire you. It is a privilege to accompany Gloria on her healing journey. I wish YOU, the reader, self-knowledge and vibrant health in all aspects of your being.

Dr. Sonia Telfer, BSc. (Hons.) MD CCFP FCFP
Family Physician

PREFACE

How I Dealt with Cancer in a Non-Conventional Way came about as a result of my diagnosis with breast cancer and the discovery made from it as to how fearfully and wonderfully made we are. It exposes our wonderfully-made body and emphasizes the role our Creator plays in our life.

How I Dealt with Cancer in a Non-Conventional Way encourages you to think for yourself, to do your own research and to take charge of your life instead of giving it over to someone else. It is about enlightenment, empowerment and responsibility. It explains that your body can heal itself and lists some of the things used from my arsenal against the diagnosis of cancer and why each is necessary for healing. There are two methods used for exorcising cancer – the conventional way and the non-conventional way. I chose the non-conventional way.

At the time in which I grew up, medicine was not in the form of tablets but in the form of "bush medicine", meaning that for every ailment there was an herb used for healing. For example, a poultice was used to remove poisons from the body. One could have felt the pulling sensation as they drew the poison out. Some were made from fresh aloe leaves which were heated, cut down the middle and applied to boils or swellings. The leaves of the castor oil plant were used in a bath to reduce swelling in the joints, and pain in the body. It was also used with stroke patients.

Packaged teas were not fashionable then. The leaves of certain plants and trees like the calabash (gourd), soursop, lime, mint and ginger were used in the making of teas. In addition to the leaves of the lime tree, the buds were also used. Drinks were made from limes, lemons, oranges and ginger.

Revelation 22: 1-2, KJV mentions in part *"and the leaves of the tree were for the healing of the nations."* This was taken seriously for that was all we knew. Being born in an era and in a part of the world where "the leaves of the tree" were used for healing made it easier for me to choose the non-conventional route instead of the conventional.

It is hoped that you will find *How I Dealt with Cancer in a Non-Conventional Way* inspirational and encouraging, and allow it to comfort you as you face your challenge for when we are challenged, we sometimes feel that we are alone.

The information in *How I Dealt with Cancer in a Non-Conventional Way* is for educational purposes and is not to be used as a medical guide. It is a sharing of how I dealt with cancer after my diagnosis. It is hoped that you will work with your doctor and health professionals if choosing the non-conventional way as I worked with mine, even though I disregarded some of her instructions. I do hope that you have a caring, understanding and compassionate doctor like mine. We laughed a lot. Laughter is a part of healing.

ACKNOWLEDGMENTS

Giving thanks always for all things unto God and
the Father in the name of our Lord Jesus Christ.
(Ephesians 3: 20, KJV)

Thanks to:

Veronica Phillips and Bibianna Remy who encouraged me to
have this book printed when I had no intention of doing so.

Victor and Maureen Greene who took time out from their
busy schedules to review this book.

Last, but by no means least, my sister Gerlyn (Erna) Austin,
who painstakingly made corrections with her left hand after
a stroke immobilized her dominant right hand.

INTRODUCTION

Beloved, think it not strange concerning the fiery
trial which is to try you, as though some strange
thing happened unto you, but rejoice…
(1 Peter 4: 12, KJV)

Cancer is on the rise and the war that is being waged against it is not working by using the old traditional ways referred to as conventional. In recognition of this, a new way is on the horizon. Awareness campaigns are being held to introduce this new way. This new way introduces us to a natural approach towards healing. This natural approach is of an holistic nature where the emotional, mental, physical and spiritual parts of the body are addressed. This is the non-conventional way.

The body was made to heal itself. We have our part to play in bringing about that healing. We were made with an immune system to keep us healthy. When it is weak, the body is not at ease and illnesses occur. Cancer is one of the illnesses that occur. It is universal. I was diagnosed with breast cancer and chose not to go the conventional way. The accepted norm in dealing with cancer is through radiation, chemotherapy and surgery. This is the conventional way of treatment and straying from it is not acceptable by some of the medical profession and members of the public.

Let us assume that you have chosen the non-conventional way as your treatment. Choosing this way is not always easy, for there will be naysayers among your doctor, co-workers, family and friends. The pressure is so strong that you wonder if you have made the right decision and you worry, worry, worry. Negative thoughts like "he or she is the doctor and knows more than I do" enter the mind, but then you conclude that it is your body and you should have control over it. You step out in faith and stick to your decision to go the non-conventional way.

How I Dealt with Cancer in a Non-Conventional Way provides the encouragement needed to accompany you on your healing journey with hope, trust, faith, dependency and courage. Chapter 3 shows you your wonderfully-made body. Chapter 2 shows how I handled the dis-ease and Chapter 6 lists natural ways to help in the restoration of your body to its former glory. Chapter 7 shows you how to develop trust and faith. These chapters helped to strengthen my resolve in light of a remark to my not going the conventional way: *"Does she want to die?"*

How I Dealt with Cancer in a Non-Conventional Way shows the love and care our Creator, God, the Universe, Source, Spirit, Our Higher Self or whatever you choose to call the one who made you has for you. He did not just make you and leave you to fend for yourself, but is with you through the good times and the bad times for you are His temple in whom He dwells. Within these pages the word Creator is mostly used to show the intimacy between you and your source of creation. In those instances, it is more meaningful than the use of the word God.

It is hoped that within the pages of *How I Dealt with Cancer in a Non-Conventional Way*, you will find the needed help and encouragement as you journey towards a cancer-free body.

ABBREVIATIONS

AHCC	Active Hexose Correlated Compound
KJV	King James Version
NIV	New International Version
NK Cells	Natural Killer Cells
NRSV	New Revised Standard Version

THE DIAGNOSIS

For misery does not come from the earth, nor does
trouble sprout from the ground; but human beings
are born to trouble just as sparks fly upwards.
(Job 5: 6-7, NRSV)

I had been taking yearly mammograms for over twenty years. One of those mammograms caused my doctor to refer me to a surgeon. Biopsies were done. It was interesting that having passed my threescore years and ten and living on borrowed time biblically, my body was diagnosed with cancer of the breast which is an abnormal growth of cells. Did this signal the end of my life?

When the surgeon told me that the "dis-ease" in my body resulted in cancer, I did not react until he mentioned the word mastectomy to which I exclaimed, *"What?"* The word mastectomy to me meant "final." He said it very calmly as though he was saying "Let's go for a walk." What he was telling me was that I had two breasts and soon I would be having one. That was unacceptable. Another appointment was scheduled. At that time I was to be accompanied by a family member. Throughout the ordeal it never entered my mind to ask myself the question, *"Why me?"* for had I done so, I would have been pointing my finger at someone else. Why would I wish this "dis-ease" of the body on anyone?

Throughout my seventy-odd years, I came to realize that life is like a seesaw going up and down, and like the seesaw, our life could be up one minute and down the next. That we cannot change, but we can change the way we look at it and the way we handle it. When I went to the hospital, I was on top of the seesaw for the thought of mastectomy never entered my mind. I was hopeful that the results would be positive, but when I got the results, I was down at the bottom, which did not last long. How I looked at my life then was not with hopelessness, but with hope for the seesaw always goes back up.

The seesaw is indiscriminate. Everyone rides upon it. It has no respect for social position, wealth, beauty, race, age, sex, religion or color. It is the vehicle we all use to take us towards unfurling. Instead of asking the question, "Why me?" it should be "Why not me?" The word "mastectomy" shocked me so much that it never occurred to me to ask that question of myself. It was my turn to be at the bottom of the seesaw, but I knew the seesaw never remains at the bottom; it always goes back up. There is always someone at the top who will send you back up when you are at the bottom.

Perhaps I knew this instinctively which was why I did not worry and why I had hope.

It is general knowledge that every person has cancer cells in the body. They are to be feared, for they create havoc within the body. There are different reasons given for the cause of cancer, some of which are exposure to chemicals in the environment; non-release of old hurts and resentments from the past which are referred to as cellular memories which sap our energy leaving us vulnerable; heredity; lifestyle choices; cells growing out of control; mold; lack of Vitamin D; low oxygen in the body's cells; lack of proper energy flow; excess estrogen in our food and water; mucus; and in the case of breast cancer – underwire bra, iodine deficiency; lack of magnesium; and on and on it continues as more discoveries are made.

Cancer cells feed on mucus. Some foods like dairy products, wheat products, refined carbohydrates and dried foods cause mucus because of an allergic reaction to these foods.

The over-use of the oils and fats or trans-fat in fried foods stimulates the production of mucus. When we say, *"I have a frog in my throat,"* I wonder if the frog is not mucus. I loved fried foods and still do, especially fried fish. Some things were hard for me to give up and fried fish was one of them. Raw fruits and vegetables are excellent mucus cleansers as they supply nutrients for healing, rejuvenation and the replacement of old cells with new ones.

Bacteria in the body can use sugar for food, thus weakening the immune system. The Creator of my fearfully and wonderfully-made body did not just create me and leave me to fend for myself. It provided me with an immune system – the tool needed to protect myself against disease and keep me healthy. When the immune system is strong, it fights off diseases and infections. When it is weak, illnesses like cancer occur. The immune system is the body's defense against invaders such as infectious organisms. Its system is made up of cells, tissues and organs whose job is to protect the body making it immune to bacteria. Mucus is associated with the respiratory system, the gastrointestinal tract, and the lymphatic system. Excess mucus creates a feeding ground for viruses.

These causes create a breakdown of the immune system. Cancer cells, present in our bodies, are kept in control by a special immune cell, NK. When this is weak, whether from old age, poor nutrition or stress, the cells multiply with nothing to hold them in check. Cancer cells supposedly thrive on solid foods but many people eat solid foods and do not have cancer, so what activates them in some and not in others? I did wonder what activated them in me and some questions surfaced:

Did I bring it about?

Did it have anything to do with my way of thinking?

Was my Creator trying to tell me something? If so, what?

What changes did I need to make in my life?

Women are told to check their breasts for lumps. We are even taught how to do it. I wonder if this does not create a fear in us which can lead to the development of a lump which we search for, month after month. We associate a lump in the breast with cancer, therefore being urged to search for a lump would create fear. Our reasoning is "A lump is supposed to be there, that is why the powers that be are telling me to look for one. I had better produce it."

Why do we think there must be one? In our minds, cancer means mastectomy and death. Isn't there a softer, kinder, more humane way of dealing with the detection of breast cancer than the known way?

There are many different types of cancer – breast, prostate, lung, ovarian, mouth, throat, etc., etc. It seems as though there is one for every part of the body because these cells are everywhere and are not localized. Yet, the Psalmist praised his Creator, for the design of his body. "I will praise thee, for I am *"fearfully and wonderfully made,"* (Psalms 139: 14, KJV).

Random acts do happen and *"time and chance happens to us all"*. These random acts of time and chance test our faith. The test of faith is not when things are going good, it is when they are not. This is when we exercise faith. It is also the time when we wonder if our Creator has not abandoned us. This is the time we wonder where He is with the promises He made about never leaving us or forsaking us and always being our friend. We reason that friends do not abandon friends in time of need.

The Apostle James tells us that when we face trials (these random acts of time and chance) of any kind, to consider them nothing but pure joy because it is the testing of our faith which produces endurance. Though we would rather not have them, these random acts of time and chance enable us to unfurl like rolled-up flags so that what we are, wonderful and lovingly-made people, can be revealed. The challenges bring about the unfurling. No challenges, no unfurling. In hindsight we realize that what James says is true. He spoke Truth.

Suffering is an attention-getter. It is our greatest teacher. We learn from our suffering something which would reveal more of ourselves to us. Not one of us can go through life unscathed. But, when the challenges do come and come they will, we each like to know that there is someone who can hold our hand. Look beyond the appearance of the challenge to the One who is waiting on the other side of the valley in which you find yourself, to the One who is willing and ready to help. The One you are waiting for is your Creator. Challenges build strength and faith to cope with life's adversities.

When we are being pruned, we ask the question, *"Why me?"* without realizing that we are not the only one being pruned, and that sometime or other pruning takes place in everyone's life. A gardener knows that if he/she wants his/her trees to produce more fruits, he/she has to prune them. The question to be asked is not, "Why me?" but "Why? Why did the incident occur? What transformational changes are necessary?"

Though pruning is painful, adopt a positive attitude towards it. When we prune our trees and they bring forth more fruit, we are pleased. So it is when we are pruned and bring forth more fruit, the world becomes a better place in which to live as we bring forth fruits of love, joy, peace, longsuffering, gentleness, goodness, faith and meekness (not weakness). The world needs more of this. One of the fruits that resulted from my pruning was compassion. Hopefully the world is a better place because of it. When we plant a garden, we nurture it, take care to remove weeds, bugs, water, fertilize and remove dead plants. I realized I took better care of my garden than I took of myself.

CHAPTER 1

GOLDEN APPLES

A word fitly spoken is like apples of
gold in pictures of silver.
(Proverbs 25: 11, KJV)

1. Cancer cells feed on mucus.
2. Dairy products, wheat products, refined carbohydrates and dried foods cause mucus.
3. Bacteria can use sugar for food.
4. The immune system is the body's defense against invaders.
5. Raw fruits and vegetables are excellent mucus cleansers.
6. Cancer cells are kept in control by a special immune cell – NK.
7. Peace comes from within.
8. It takes time and courage to develop faith.
9. Trust and Faith are necessary tools in a challenge.
10. We learn from our suffering something which would reveal more of ourselves.
11. Time and chance happens to us all. They test our faith.
12. The state of being perfect results in love.
13. Challenges build strength and faith to cope with life's adversities.

HANDLING THE DIS-EASE

No testing has overtaken you that is not common to
everyone. God is faithful, and he will not let you be tested
beyond your strength, but with the testing he will also
provide the way out so that you may be able to endure it.
(1 Corinthians 10: 13, NRSV)

A disease of the body means that it is not at ease, it is under
stress. Notice how relaxed regiments are when told to stand
at ease, how lose and limber the body is when compared to
the order to stand at attention. Notice how stiff and tense
the body is then? My body was not at ease.

When we are at the bottom of the seesaw, the words
quoted by those who are at the top "God does not give us
more than we can bear," are not words of comfort when
we are wondering why would He give us anything that

is painful to bear. In looking at the last part of the verse however, *"he will also provide the way out so that you may be able to endure it,"* we see loving arms eager to enfold us, to comfort us and strengthen us.

I was asked by the surgeon if anyone in the family had cancer. The answer was "Yes." A cousin, a sister and an aunt died after being diagnosed with it. Was this my fate too? I chose not to believe it. I absolutely refused to give cancer any power at all over me. It is not a good thing to inherit and I had no intention of claiming that inheritance.

Upon arriving home from the hospital after knowing the results of the biopsy, the first thing I did was to research the dis-ease from books and the Internet. What would we do without the Internet? The information found therein backed up my belief that the body can heal itself. Mother Nature made us and she can and will take care of us. She provided everything needed for our health: fruits, vegetables, water, and fresh air. It is our choice as to whether or not we use them and how we use them.

Throughout the research, the recurring thought in my mind was, "When I cut myself I do nothing to the cut and it heals, so why can't my body heal this dis-ease too? There has to be something or someone inside of me that does the healing." Armed with information, I devised a plan of action. I was determined to prove that my body can heal itself if given the right nutrients. In the back of my mind I heard the words, *"Prove me now herewith, saith the Lord of hosts, if I will not open you the windows of heaven, and pour you out a blessing, that there shall not be room enough to receive it* (Malachi 3: 10, KJV)." This sentence was drummed into me from my earlier church days.

An opportunity presented itself for me to pick up the challenge. I accepted. From the information gathered, I created a new me and did things that previously I was much too busy to do. Isn't it interesting that we never have time to do the things we know we should do until something happens to cause us to face ourselves? The new me exercised, watched what I ate, sat out in the sun, rested, took afternoon naps and went to bed early.

According to my research, my diet was to be fruits and vegetables which I seldom ate, so I emptied my refrigerator and kitchen cupboard of meats, tinned foods, eggs, sugar, oils and whatever else my research said I should not eat. It was heartbreaking since I had bought some of the foodstuff a few days before the diagnosis.

Someone told me about the Budwig Breakfast Diet of cottage cheese, honey, flaxseed oil, flaxseed and fruits which I began using. The cottage cheese should have been organic, but as I was unaware of this, I used the ones sold in the grocery stores. Although I had stopped using dairy products, the combination sounded good to me and after my first taste, there was no turning back. Apparently, organic cottage cheese has sulfur proteins. The combination with the flaxseed oil makes the oil water soluble and thus is easily absorbed into the cells.

Perhaps my ignorance of not having the right type of cottage cheese did no harm to my body because I took the breakfast mixture in faith. It was most enjoyable. An added benefit was that the flaxseed and flaxseed oil made it into a type of detox. I alternated the Budwig Breakfast with smoothies made with apples, bananas, carrots, any of the berries and/or any other fruit that is in season, to which is added ground flaxseeds, honey and cinnamon. Using a blender is better than a juicer for the juicer separates the juice from the fiber. We need the fiber to help with digestion.

Lunch was a raw salad of broccoli, cauliflower, patchoi, tomatoes, lettuce, onions, garlic, herbs and cooked dried beans. The only oils used for cooking was olive oil and for salads, flax oil. My stomach shrunk so much that the evening meal was a cup of green tea. I was very hungry until my body got accustomed to its new diet. After a while lunch became very boring, so that when I went visiting, I cheated and ate whatever was placed in front of me.

I consumed no dairy products other than the grocery-bought cottage cheese which I thought I was supposed to use, fried foods or alcohol. I cut out sugar completely. This is not quite true. There are different types of sugar – sucrose, fructose and glucose. Sucrose is refined sugar like table sugar, fructose is the natural sugar in fruits and glucose is sugar in the blood. My sugar came from fruits. I used sea salt instead of the iodized table salt. What I missed most of all from my diet were fried fish and ice cream. I loved both and was therefore surprised at the ease with which I gave them up. I was determined to "Prove me now herewith" to see whether the blessing of healing would have descended upon me.

I avoided saying, *"I have cancer."* I did not own it as it was not something good that I wanted. I disarmed it by saying *"I was diagnosed with cancer."* Perhaps you are asking "What is the difference in the phrasing, it's all the same." This is the difference: I have a physical body and a spiritual body. The physical body was diagnosed with cancer. The spiritual body was not. If cancer were a good thing, people would rejoice instead of expressing horror when they hear that someone has been diagnosed with it. A friend e-mailed me that she shed a tear when she heard about my diagnosis. She probably saw it as a death sentence.

It is important not to give the dis-ease a name. Giving the dis-ease of the body a name conjures up in the mind the stigma attached to it. Rather, think of it as a malfunction of the body. In thinking this way, your attitude will be to get the body functioning again. This removes the *"woe is me"* attitude and waiting passively for someone to tell you what to do as you give your life over to them. Take action! Do your own research! What may work for one person may not work for you. Everyone's immune system is different.

Do not identify with the cancer. You are not it and it is not you. If you are not comfortable with conventional treatment, then research alternatives. There are many alternatives called "Protocols" that are being bandied about. A non-conventional protocol can include vitamins, herbs, exercise, spices, and whatever natural things that can help the body return to wholeness. Water is usually included, but the water to be drunk should be purified or filtered water, but depending on the part of the world in which one lives, purified or filtered water is not always available.

I forced myself to drink eight glasses of water. I thought I was doing great until I heard somewhere that it should be ten. I never made it to ten. I had no access to purified or filtered water and used rain water which fell from the sky into my containers. I collected rain water from the spout on my roof until I realized that the water could be contaminated from the dust and leaves which collected there.

I read of and used a new natural treatment which involved the stimulation of the immune system so that tumors are destroyed by the NK cells. This treatment is derived from a substance found in certain Japanese mushrooms called Active Hexose Correlated Compound or AHCC in capsule form. It is supposed to increase the natural killer (NK) cells. Is this a wonder "natural" drug? It is supposed to provide extra power to help the body fight the cancer as its primary function is the strengthening of the immune system. It is also supposed to act as a deterrent against any disease.

I took action against the dis-ease by doing the research into it. When you take action, you feel powerful. Fear masks power. Get rid of the fear and the power emerges. Remember, we were not given *a spirit of fear but of power and a sound mind;* a sound mind to have the courage to take the necessary action. Once we decide to take action and step out, things happen.

We are afraid of what we do not understand. I decided to research this dis-ease of the body, and in doing so, I now have knowledge which I would not have had otherwise. With knowledge comes wisdom. The wisdom gained from the knowledge has taught me that there is nothing to fear but fear itself.

Fear paralyzes and prevents us from taking action, but fear should propel us into taking action. Our beliefs influence our mind which influences our body. Our beliefs can limit us or expand us. Beliefs create emotions which create feelings. Our belief creates our reality. We have the power to create. What we can create are healthy healing thoughts. We attract to ourselves what we are thinking about. This can make us or break us. Looking beyond the appearance of the dis-ease and seeing ourselves healthy, creates healing.

The feel of your body or what we call our "gut feeling," will tell you when you have made a right decision. If you feel comfort, it is right; if discomfort, your decision is wrong. Radiation and/or chemotherapy had to seem right to me for me to use them and since they did not, I decided not to use either. The feel of your body should also be used in the choice of medication; treatment and diet for no two persons are alike. What may be good for the persons you read or hear about, may not be good for you. Decide your own treatment and diet by the feelings in your body.

Choosing to "prove me now herewith," I kept the words *"I am fearfully and wonderfully made; nothing is growing in my fearfully and wonderfully-made body,"* in the forefront of my mind. It has always been my belief that nothing should grow in my body, no lumps or tumors for if it is the temple of my Creator, there was not enough room for Him and the lumps and tumors.

Prayer and meditation were also a great help. I never managed to do the meditation the way the instructors said it should be done. My meditation was mindless as I sat with eyes closed for about fifteen minutes watching what came in and out of my mind, feeling my feelings. My prayer was simple: "Thy Will be done." Death did not enter my mind as being a part of that Will. My Creator's Will for me was not any form of suffering. A Will is a written legal document for the disposal of property after death. It can also mean intention, purpose and/or desire and is usually an instrument of great joy. When a Will is left to an heir or heirs it has to be probated. Monies have to be paid to probate it before the proceeds of the Will, outlining the person's intentions, desires and/or purpose, can be fulfilled.

For the Will of my Creator to be probated, faith was the currency needed. "Whatever you ask for in prayer with faith, you will receive" (Matthew 21: 22, NRSV). My prayer ended with an act of faith by giving thanks. This sealed the prayer as it said, "I know that whatever I ask for is already granted for, before I called, you answered."

Having a large flower garden was a great help, for I sat in it on mornings when the sun was at its highest and watched the birds and butterflies as they flitted around. When I felt I had enough sun, I moved inside and listened to soothing music. Resting is very important. Your body knows when it needs to do so. Listen and obey. I found it important to live my life as normally as possible so I continued doing what I had been doing before diagnosis. I tended my garden, shopped, prepared meals, sewed, entertained, visited friends and family, exercised, wrote newsletters and volunteered at an early childhood center.

I found tending a kitchen garden to be very therapeutic. You do not need a plot of land to do gardening. A "kitchen garden" can be made out of pots, dark-colored heavyweight plastic bags or any other containers in which you can plant herbs like mint, shallots, celery, basil, chives, dill, garlic, oregano, marjoram, tarragon, sage, turmeric and thyme, all of which are useful in the fight against cancer. Tomatoes and lettuce also grow well in pots. Label the pots so that you know what is planted where. If you are using pots, plastic bags or containers, make sure there are holes in the bottom for drainage of water when you wet them. Tending a kitchen garden will relax you. Notice how you feel when gathering the materials for planting. Challenged? Excited? How do you feel when harvesting? Empowered? How do you feel when using your produce? Accomplished? Fulfilled?

If you have access to a plot of land for gardening, you will need soil, manure, irrigation and other things. Check out the library, bookstore or Internet for information on how to make a kitchen garden or a garden. According to the part of the world you are in, watch out for the birds. They love the tomatoes and peppers. I make a shelter for the tomatoes and peppers covering it with netting so that the water and sunlight can still penetrate. The netting falls to the ground enclosing the tomatoes and peppers. The shelter has to be sealed to prevent the birds from entering. They are very clever. I place stones all around the net on the ground. My reaped tomatoes and peppers are whole.

CHAPTER 2

GOLDEN APPLES

A word fitly spoken is like apples of
gold in pictures of silver.
(Proverbs 25: 11, KJV)

1. Do not give the disease a name.
2. Everyone's immune system is different.
3. Do not identify with the cancer.
4. We have the power to create.
5. A disease of the body means that it is not at ease.
6. Get rid of fear and power emerges.
7. With knowledge comes wisdom.
8. Our belief creates our reality.

CHAPTER 3

MY WONDERFULLY-MADE BODY

I will praise thee for I am fearfully and
wonderfully made, marvelous are thy works
and that my soul knoweth right well.
(Psalms 139: 14, KJV)

In my research into the disease, I was amazed at my discoveries, one of which was how fearfully and wonderfully made I am. Understanding how the body is made and the part it plays in its dis-ease can remove fear of any dis-ease.

The body's cells have their own intelligence as they communicate with one another. They can change themselves into any type of cell if needed and they know how to heal. Before an immune cell secretes any cancer-fighting agent, it has to identify the existence of cancer cells. It uses messengers called T-cells to notify the rest of the immune system to activate itself and produce cells to kill the cancer cells. The body tags the cancer cells to be destroyed, to prevent the killer cells from wiping out the wrong ones. How does the body know to do all this? What is the body? Who lives in the body? Think about it.

Have you ever heard of apoptosis? It is the death of cells. This is the method the body uses to destroy these cells. Cells signal their own termination to keep the body's natural process of cell division in check. Those that are damaged or infected remove themselves from the body through apoptosis without harming other cells. The cells reduce in size and break down into fragments enclosed in membranes so as not to harm nearby cells.

The body heals itself. When we cut ourselves, the cut heals by itself. Why cannot the body heal itself of this malfunction – cancer? Is it that where the cut is concerned we do not think about it because we expect it to heal, that our mind is not involved, or we take it for granted, but where cancer is concerned, our mind is involved with fear of the disease, fear of death?

The word "cancer" puts fear into our hearts because we associate it with death. In years past, it used to be hush-hush as though just the mention of the word made the dis-ease contagious and shameful. We create our fear of it, but fear is an illusion which masks our power. Life is power, not fear. We should not look upon cancer as a death sentence, but as an opportunity to know our body which is *fearfully and wonderfully made.*

This is how *fearfully and wonderfully made* our body is. It is made up of several parts which perform different functions. For example, the kidneys are trash collectors.

They collect leftovers from the food that the body does not need after it extracts what it needs for energy and repair of itself. What do you think would happen if the kidneys did not remove this waste? The body would not be able to function as properly as it should. It attends to its own needs. It repairs itself. It thinks and acts on its own. It moves itself from place to place. It regulates its body temperature.

Created in the image and likeness of our Creator, our fearfully and wonderfully-made body has Godlike qualities. It communicates. It is the temple of our Creator. It is holy. Know your body. It is wise. Be aware of what is taking place within and without. Know how each part feels. Co-operate with it. Learn to love your body and the parts that make it up. See your body as being whole as it is. You were fearfully and wonderfully made. Knowing yourself helps you to make better choices. Knowing myself helped in my choice of the non-conventional way. Knowing our body gives us power.

We have the power to heal our bodies. Get past the emotion of fear. We generate our own fears. We do not create our fears only in the now, but also into the future. Fear plagues us constantly, so we prepare ourselves for some disasters that might happen. When we fear, we worry.

We make ourselves sick from worrying when we are afraid and without realizing it, our attitude of worrying is saying that the all-powerful Creator is not powerful enough to work out what we are afraid of. This is not true. He did not place the spirit of fear within us. We do that on our own. Our minds are not sound when we are fearful. We allow ourselves to be obsessed day and night by thoughts which enter our minds. This unsound mind is harmful to our health and peace. He gave us power, love and a sound mind.

We have to surrender our fears before we can have the power, love and sound mind. We have to be unconcerned about the things we are fearful about, knowing that everything is alright. We need to realize our fears do not make sense and need to be examined to find the root cause. We worry because we cannot see the way out of our predicament, challenge or trouble. We worry because we are afraid. We are afraid because we cannot see beyond the appearance. We try comforting each other with the words, *"Don't worry"* but these words mean nothing to you who are in a maze and who cannot see or find a way out.

In being fearful, we are creating and giving life to our creation that there is a power greater than our Creator who can withhold and who is withholding our good from us. Even though we may know countless key verses of trust and repeat them one after the other, we still worry. Our worrying is made worse by the fact that we know we should not worry and so we worry that we are worrying. We worry because we have not yet attained the level of conscious trust necessary to not worry. As we grow more in conscious trust, we worry less and less and understand more and more that we were not given a spirit of fear, but of power.

Consciousness is the realization of your true self - a vessel in whom the Spirit of your Creator lives. This realization helps us to see that we have in us the spirit of power and not of fear. Having the consciousness causes us to let go and let it do its work for *"It is the Father, living in me, who is doing His work."* We have been given power and self-control to conquer fear. It takes time to recognize this power and to use it.

Though it is difficult to understand how we can have peace when circumstances say differently, glimmers of light appear to us from time to time to show us that it is possible. The day will come when we will be able to see beyond appearances. On that day, we will have replaced our worry with our trust and be like the fowls (birds) of the air "for they sow not, neither do they reap, nor gather into barns; yet your heavenly Father feedeth them..." The question is then asked "are ye not much better than they" (Matthew 6: 26, KJV)? The birds of the air worry about nothing for they know that there is someone to take care of their needs.

To overcome fear is our biggest challenge. It blocks our good as it sets up a barrier which limits the good we desire. It destroys our happiness and is the result of a lack of faith in the One for whom nothing is impossible. To help in overcoming our fears, we must remember that we are a part of the Divine, the temple in whom He lives. With this knowing, who and what is there to fear? Faith does not come overnight, but is built little by little.

We must convert our fear into faith. We must have the confidence that no matter whatever happens, everything is alright because there is someone bigger than us, someone who cares enough, someone who takes pleasure in giving us the kingdom. We should accept this gift not by fearing, but by loving for *"Perfect love casts out fear."* Love for the One who knows nothing of limitation and is the Source of all things, will cast out fear.

I was re-watching an old documentary on our creation recently. I was awe-struck to see the coming together of the egg and sperm and the result of it – a fearfully and wonderfully-made body. Watching the fetus grow until it was ready to be born was spellbinding. I thought whoever or whatever came up with the design was not human and had to be held in awe. I imagined myself as that baby being conceived and born, having nothing to do with my creation.

Understanding the process of my creation made me look at myself differently. The baby created its own immune system separate from its mother's immune system and encased it. Did it not do so, the mother's immune system would have taken it for a foreign invader and destroyed it. The immune system would have been doing its job, for that is what it is supposed to do – protect the body from invaders.

The fetus has the wisdom to know the value of the immune system and creates its own so as not to be taken for a foreign invader by its mother's immune system because it wants to live. This showed me that I too must protect myself from the foreign invaders of cancer cells by having a strong immune system because I, too, want to live. The key to the obliteration of foreign invaders then, is in the strengthening of the immune system. I saw then why the Psalmist praised his Creator for his fearfully and wonderfully-made body. If my body is wonderfully and fearfully made, is the dis-ease of cancer an illusion? Yes and No. Yes, it is an illusion for my spiritual body. No, it is not an illusion for my physical body. It is real.

The Psalmist praised his Creator for being fearfully and wonderfully made yet it is an accepted fact that every person has cancer cells. If we are fearfully and wonderfully made, why do we have cancer cells which are not an enhancement to the body but a detriment? Shouldn't the accepted fact be that every person has cells, some of which become cancerous when we do not maintain the body? What do you think?

CHAPTER 3

GOLDEN APPLES

A word fitly spoken is like apples of
gold in pictures of silver.
(Proverbs 25: 11, KJV)

1. The body's cells have their own intelligence.
2. Apoptosis is the death of cells.
3. The body heals itself.
4. It is the temple of our Creator.
5. It is holy.
6. We generate our fears.
7. We worry because we are afraid.
8. Overcoming fear is our biggest challenge.
9. Our beliefs influence our mind which influence our body.
10. The body regulates its own body temperature and removes its own waste.
11. Consciousness is the realization of your true self – a vessel in which the Spirit of your Creator lives.

CHAPTER 4

THOUGHTS

For he that wavereth is like a wave of the sea driven
with the wind and tossed for let not that man
think that he shall receive any thing of the Lord. A
double minded man is unstable in all his ways.
(James 1: 6-8, KJV)

One of the functions of my wonderfully made body is to think. That function has to be carefully watched, for thoughts seem to have a mind of their own. They are either negative or positive and can either make us or break us. They are powerful things and can work for or against us. They can create fear, anger and emotional stress. Even though we think positively, negative thoughts come creeping in.

My sister who has passed her threescore years and ten (70) expects to be looked after because, as she puts it, she is old. Since we live within a stone's throw of each other, it is her expectation that I look after her. There was a great temptation not to do all that I could to restore my health, to just give in by doing nothing, so that she would not lean on me. She has no aches, pains or diseases, but in her mind, I should be caring for her.

The temptation was great to just give up on myself, for I saw her dependency on me as a burden which I did not need, but realized that anger, bitterness and resentment were detrimental to my health, and it was important that they be removed from my thoughts. I could not afford to be double-minded in my way of thinking, one minute wanting to be healed and the next minute not wanting to, so that she would not lean on me. I had to decide whether or not I wanted healing. The decision was made in favor of healing.

Mention is made of my sister, not to denigrate, but to show how we can allow others to influence our state of mind by not doing the best we can for ourselves in challenging situations like dealing with the diagnosis of cancer. Right thinking purifies us. Being double-minded and" like a wave of the sea driven by the wind and tossed" to and fro does not create peace within the body. Even so, it was not easy for me to give up my anger and resentment. I had to find something with which to replace it. I found the lost love I had for my sister as memories of the good times we had growing up came flooding back from time to time. By giving up my anger and resentment what I was demonstrating was forgiveness. Who knows how many times she forgave me for things I did to her that I was unaware of?

We determine the type of life we have by the choices we make. We make the choices we do by the way we think.

There is always something or someone we blame for the situation we are in, whether it is we ourselves, someone else, or God. Until we forgive whoever we think is responsible, we cannot move on. My choice was to forgive her for her way of thinking because her way of thinking was fear-based. When we are fear-based, self-centeredness is usually at the bottom of the fear, for our thoughts do not allow us to think of anyone but ourselves.

Forgiveness is the key to moving on. Without it we are stuck in the time of the event. The incident may be over, but we relive it over and over again, bringing it back to life. Life moves forward daily, continually evolving, and so must we. To forgive is to use a double-edged sword to show mercy, not only to the one who has hurt us, but also to ourselves. When we do not forgive, we are the ones who suffer the most. A lack of forgiveness causes us to have unhealthy thoughts which can lead to destruction of the mind and body. The longer we take to forgive, the reason for not forgiving becomes more distorted.

Hanging on to the past drains us of energy, of strength, of power. It is difficult for the mind and the body to live in two worlds at the same time – the past and the present. This creates instability. *"A double-minded man is unstable in all his ways."* For the sake of sanity, peace of mind, health, the past must be given up. It must be forgiven and forgotten if healing is to take place. Holding on to the past robs us of life. Forgiveness, if and when we are ready to embrace it, will take time, but by moving forward one step at a time, it can and will be accomplished.

We have within us the power to forgive, the power to move on. We can hold on to hate for so long that it becomes a part of us. As such, we are afraid to give it up because we have nothing with which to replace it. The first step in growing anything is to plant a seed. For us to move on we have to take the first step by planting the seed of forgiveness. As this seed grows, our heart begins to soften. We now think and look at things differently. When this happens, we have moved on.

By moving on, we have left the old behind, and are ready for the new. We have been renewed. We have been born again. To be born again is to look forward and not backward. It is to drop the baggage of hurts and hang-ups that we carry around with us. It is to forgive. We have forgiven those who have hurt us or who we think have hurt us. We have been born anew, invigorated, ready to create a new person. We have looked beyond the appearance of what is. The old structures are broken down and new ones built.

You may be wondering how this chapter on thoughts and forgiveness helps with the dealing of cancer in a non-conventional way. Our thoughts control us. They control whether or not we forgive. Life is a choice. We determine the type of life we have by the choices we make. We make the choices we do by the way we think. We have the right to choose what we want to experience. Why not choose healing through forgiveness?

When we do not forgive, our body is not at ease, thus it is not healthy holding unforgiving thoughts towards anyone, including ourselves. A great weight is placed upon the body which weakens it and makes it impossible to move on. By removing this load, we are free to concentrate on the healing of the body without any hindrance. We need a clear mind in order to deal with the diagnosis of cancer. Jesus showed that forgiveness is a necessary part of healing, for when he saw the palsied man lying on a bed he forgave him his sins "and he arose, and departed to his house." As we too forgive others the real or imagined wrongs they do to us, we too will have our bodies functioning again.

CHAPTER 4

GOLDEN APPLES

"A word fitly spoken is like apples of
gold in pictures of silver."
(Proverbs 25: 11, KJV)

1. Forgiveness is the key to moving on.
2. To forgive is to show mercy to the one who has hurt us and to our self.
3. The longer we take to forgive, the reason for not forgiving becomes more distorted.
4. Hanging on to the past drains us of energy, of strength, of power.
5. To be born again is to look forward and not backward.
6. We determine the type of life we have by the choices we make.
7. We make the choices we do by the way we think.
8. Our thoughts seem to have a mind of their own.

CHAPTER 5

UNDER CONSTANT SCRUTINY

"What is man that you make so much of him, that you give him so much attention, that you examine him every morning and test him every moment? Will you never look away from me, or let me alone even for an instant?"
(Job 7: 17-19, NIV)

One does not expect to be diagnosed with cancer in one's senior years. We expect the senior years to be the time to review life, when we complement ourselves that we have made it so far through the turbulence of life and can now look forward to enjoyment before the lifespan expires.

This is the time we are ready to do things we were not able to do because of work, raising a family, or whatever else prevented us from doing so, and then wham, one is diagnosed with cancer. We looked forward to contributing to the world. Whenever I heard of someone in their 60's, 70's, 80's or 90's being diagnosed with cancer, I was puzzled. My 80-odd year old aunt was diagnosed with cancer and I just could not understand why, at that time. Why would anyone in that age group be diagnosed with cancer? What happened? What caused it? Surely by that age we should be exempt from cancer.

Since being diagnosed with cancer, I understand that it is a dis-ease of the body, and as time and chance happens to all, no age group is exempt from the body's not being at ease. The seesaw is indiscriminate. Was my diagnosis a misfortune? The word misfortune implies that one has missed a fortune. Fortune is described as a hypothetical force that governs the events of one's life, wealth or riches. It is assumed that there is something or someone that is doing the governing of the events which take place in one's life.

If this is so, is that something or someone responsible for the dis-ease of my body? My answer would have to be No. I am responsible for the state of my body. Did I think I was under constant scrutiny? No. I should have been the one to put myself under constant scrutiny and not allow my body to be out of ease.

The dis-ease of my body was a fortune because of the knowledge gained about the make-up and workings of my wonderfully-made body. The something or someone played a part in my healing, for I did not make the vegetables, fruits and other non-conventional things I used to bring it about. Like Job, I could have questioned my Creator about being under constant scrutiny, but I was too concerned with what had caused this dis-ease so late in my life.

Facing the detection of cancer is not an easy challenge to cope with, more so detection in someone in their senior years living alone. Who prepares the meals? Who takes you to the doctor's office? Who does the laundry? Who offers comfort? Who does the shopping? Who does the cleaning? Who does the banking? Who does whatever needs to be done? Are there organizations dealing with senior cancer patients who live alone?

This is where family and friends can make a difference. When we are in a challenge, it is comforting for our family and friends to share in it. They help to carry the load. If we do not share, we are robbing them of expressing love. Being aware of someone else's challenge takes us out of our self-centeredness, as our attention is placed on the other person. Our life's purpose is one of service. It is love.

My sister who expected me to take care of her developed a stroke. She had no family of her own, so I became the caregiver. It was not easy looking after her and myself. When it became too difficult I hired a nurse for her. She passed away six months later. I was relieved that she was gone, but did not feel guilty, for before the stroke, she looked forward to death. She was not afraid of it. Perhaps that is why the duration of the stroke was only six months, while for some, the duration is years.

Twenty months before my diagnosis and my older sister's passing away from her stroke, another sister suffered a stroke on her right side. I was the caregiver. She did recover her speech and a limited use of her right hand and foot and returned to her home three months later.

I felt like Job and could have said "What am I that you make so much of me, that you give me so much attention, that you examine me every morning and test me every moment? Will you never look away from me or let me alone even for an instant?" but I did not, having read about the good things that resulted from his constant scrutiny.

I did not share my journey with many as it was something I wanted to take on my own, but called upon one or two friends when help was needed. I wanted to go through it largely on my own, for I did not want to depend too much on anyone. I wanted to discover who and what I was, as the opinion I had of myself had an impact on my life. Who was I? I was and am divine because my Creator lived and lives in me. He created my wonderful body as a vessel in which to live. I chose to believe this. I discovered that I was the temple of my Creator with His Spirit dwelling in me. I was made in His image. If I were a temple in whom He dwelled, there would not be room enough for a growth in my body and for Him. Knowing my true identity gave me the courage to persevere with my non-conventional treatment.

A friend sent me the meaning of the word courage:

Courage is standing up for your beliefs when you are threatened by those who are deceived. In other words, she was encouraging me to stick to my decision of non-conventional treatment and not to listen to the conventionalists, whoever they might have been.

CHAPTER 5

GOLDEN APPLES

A word fitly spoken is like apples of
gold in pictures of silver.
(Proverbs 25: 11, KJV)

1. We are the receptacle for our Creator's Spirit.
2. Support and encouragement strengthen us to go on.
3. Our life's purpose is one of service.
4. To serve means to help, to assist, to go out of one's way, going that extra mile.
5. Service is good works. It is love.
6. No age group is exempt from cancer.

CHAPTER 6

NON-CONVENTIONAL ARSENAL

Once a disease has entered the body, parts which
are healthy must fight it not one alone, but all.
Because a disease might mean their common
death. Nature knows this and Nature attacks the
disease with whatever help she can muster.
(Paracelsus)

An arsenal is a place where weapons and ammunitions are
stored. This chapter mentions some of them which can be
used in the war against cancer. Nature musters help from
the following non-conventional arsenal:

Raw Food: Apparently, the way our bodies react to
foreign invaders is the same way in which it reacts to cooked
foods, hence the recommendation for raw foods. They
release more white blood cells.

Our food should be our medicine, but between 30 to 85% of its nutrition is destroyed in cooking, so says one research. Fresh, raw foods have the highest levels of enzymes which promote life. Enzymes are needed by minerals and vitamins to reach the cells. Alas, our soil is deficient in minerals that are needed for our health, which makes our body suitable for bacteria, viruses and parasites.

When eating raw foods with cooked foods, the immune response is neutral. Since the body absorbs what it needs from raw foods, some experts say our raw foods should be 80-85%, and cooked foods should be 15-20%. While raw foods build the immune system, some fruits and vegetables have nutrients that kill cancer cells and can also stop the spread of cancer. Some of these foods are carrots, broccoli, cabbage, Brussels sprouts, cauliflower, peppers, asparagus, pineapple, watermelon, purple grapes, apricots and seeds, blueberries, beetroot, beets, turmeric, apples, peaches, tomatoes.

The foods listed with nutrients that kill cancer cells and that can also stop the spread of cancer are not common in every country, *"for one country is different from another, its earth is different as are its stones, wines, bread, meat and everything that grows and thrives in a specific region."* (Paracelsus) So, it does not mean that vegetables and fruits grown locally do not have healing properties just because research has not been done on them. Some of the vegetables grown in my country that are not common to North America are: breadfruit, cassava, melongene, ochro, patchoi, pigeon peas, bhaji, tannia, bodi, christophene and sim. Some of the fruits grown are: custard apple, star apple, papaw, chataigne, cashew, cherries (yellow), guava, governor plum, barbadeen, golden apple (pommecythere), sapodilla, soursop and sugar apple.

If one is to believe Genesis 1: 29, KJV which says: "And God said, Behold, I have given you every herb bearing seed, which *is* upon the face of all the earth, and every tree, in the which *is* the fruit of a tree yielding seed; to you it shall be for meat" then whatever fruits and vegetables are grown in one's country can be viewed as also having the nutrients that kill cancer cells and can also stop the spread of cancer.

Most of the fruits and vegetables listed that kill cancer cells and that can also stop the spread of cancer are found in North America, but since our Creator is no respecter of persons, surely, fruits and vegetables grown in every country will have cancer-fighting nutrients. Even so, unless we grow these ourselves or have access to where they are grown, some of the nutrients will be destroyed by the time they reach the markets or supermarkets. How many days travel before they reach us? They fill us up when eaten, but how many nutrients do they contain?

The basis for the raw food diet is taken from Genesis 1:29, KJV which says: "And God said, Behold, I have given you every herb bearing seed, which *is* upon the face of all the earth, and every tree, in the which *is* the fruit of a tree yielding seed; to you it shall be for meat." It did not say that they should not be cooked. Some of us may not be able to eat raw food. The principle behind this quote is to eat every herb bearing seed and every fruit.

Juicing is recommended for fruits or vegetables because it makes the nutrients not only more digestible but extracts more of it. More nutrients can be consumed in a shorter amount of time. I drank so much carrot juice that when I visited my doctor she was concerned by the yellowness of my palms until I told her what had caused it.

Exercise is important in the building of the immune system as well as the lymph and circulatory systems. It increases oxygen. Exercise improves our circulation, strengthens our muscles and bones. It even improves our memory, stimulates our brain and creates a feeling of well-being. It can also lengthen our life.

One of the ways to keep our body functioning as it should is through exercise. Our bodies were made to move. Have you ever noticed how many joints are in our body? They are flexible. If we do not use them, they become stiff and sore. Exercise experts say that as little as twenty minutes three times a week is sufficient to help maintain a healthy body. A common exercise is walking. Exercise helps to maintain our general health – mental, emotional, physical and spiritual.

AHCC or Active Hexose Correlated Compound is a compound derived from a mushroom used for medicinal purposes in Japan for cancer and other diseases of immune deficiency. It not only regulates the activity of several types of white blood cells, but increases the activity of natural killer cells. Natural killer cells identify abnormal cells and destroy them. It can stimulate the immune system to fight T-cells which directly attack cells taken over by cancer. Since this is not sold in my part of the world, a friend, O.B, from Canada sent it to me. I experienced no side effects.

Cancerbush known as Kankerbos by the southern Africans has been used to treat cancer for centuries. It has powerful immune boosting properties. It is a flowering plant and a relative of the pea. The leaves are used in the preparation of the tablet. I was unaware of it until my nephew, Ali, who lives in the United Kingdom and knew of it, sent it to me. Its dosage is two capsules a day. I experienced no side effects also.

Antioxidants inhibit oxidation and act as protectors for the body against the damages of free radicals. Free radicals are by-products of the chemical processes of the body which attack healthy cells, changing their DNA thus causing tumors to grow.

Selenium, an antioxidant, is a mineral found in small amounts in the body's tissues. As the body ages, selenium in the cells decreases, the immune system does not function as it should and the body becomes susceptible to disease. Some sources of selenium are grains, sunflower seeds, Brazilian nuts, onions, mushrooms, broccoli, seafood and garlic. It helps protects cells from harmful free radicals. But if taken in large amounts it can be toxic. Together selenium and Vitamin E are a team. Selenium protects within the cells and Vitamin E protects the outer cell membranes.

CoenzymeQ10 referred to as CoQ10 is an antioxidant used for the burning of oxygen within the cells which is necessary for them to do their job. It protects the body's tissues from wear and tear by destroying free radicals – unstable molecules which steal electrons at the cellular level. It also reacts with another enzyme so that cells can convert protein, fat and carbohydrates into energy.

Vitamin E, a fat-soluble vitamin (attaches to fat) found in vegetable oils, wheat germ, nuts, avocados is best taken with a meal containing some fat. There are two kinds: synthetic (dl-alpha-tocopherol) and natural (d-alpha-tocopherol). The natural kind is better absorbed and stays longer in the body than the synthetic kind. It can help in the protection of cells from damage that can lead to cancer.

Sounds have vibrations. Words have sounds. Sounds can be healing. Jesus used sound for healing in the case of the centurion's servant whom he healed by just speaking the word. Words as sounds have power to heal. "He sent his word, and healed them…" (Psalms 107: 20, KJV). Not only the words were used to heal but possibly the sound of the words, since sounds carry; they reverberate – echo and re-echo.

"He sendeth out his word, and melteth them: he causeth his wind to blow, and the waters flow" (Psalms 147: 18, KJV). The vibrational sound of the voice as the words were uttered, melted the ice, as well as causing the wind to blow and the waters to flow.

When a mother is singing her baby to sleep, it is not the words of the song, but the sound of the mother's music that causes it to sleep. The world is made up of sounds – some pleasant and some not so pleasant.

Sounds have the power to heal us, to soothe us or to have the opposite effect. When God withdrew His spirit from Saul and placed an evil spirit upon him that troubled him, his servants knew that only the sound of music could have made him well. "And it came to pass, when the evil spirit from God was upon Saul, that David took an harp, and played with his hand: so Saul was refreshed, and was well, and the evil spirit departed from him" (1 Samuel 16: 23, KJV).

As a child growing up, I remembered my mother using sound as a method of healing when our chickens were knocked out either from crossing the road and being hit by a car, or from being hit by something thrown at them. She would put a calabash (gourd) over them and pound on it, creating a sound. It appears that the vibration from the sound penetrated into their bodies, and as this penetration took place, the chickens came to life again.

Music: Just as there are types of music and songs that depress us, there are those that lift us up. Some types of music are used in healing. The cells of our bodies come alive with the right type of music. Put on some dance music and dance around. Your cells would thank you. You would make them very happy. No one to dance with? Use a broom. Whenever I have something to do and I am lazy to do so, like washing the dishes, I put on some fast-tempo music. It is amazing how the laziness disappears and how quickly the dishes are washed. Music energizes us.

Music is also used as therapy in addressing the physical, emotional, mental and spiritual challenges of individuals. It has been used as medicine for thousands of years by the ancient Greek philosophers who believed that it could heal not only the body, but the soul as well, and by Native Americans who use singing and chanting as part of their healing rituals.

I checked my music supply and selected a sound CD called *Spirit Trance* which is one from a set of CD's called *Sound Health, Sound Wealth* by Dr. Luanne Oakes. It is a one-hour CD layered with subliminal messages which I played every morning. It is a series of sounds. In this three-part set, there is also a CD which deals with healing every part of the body. It utilizes specific sound frequencies to access the body's DNA healing codes. It was also suggested that a drop of myrrh oil be placed just above the upper lip before playing the CD's. What peaceful wonderful feelings this evoked!

The sound of dripping water can be annoying at times but, if you listen attentively, the sound has a beat. One of the sounds that I enjoy listening to and which makes me feel good is the sound of raindrops on the roof. It is calming, soothing and puts a big grin on my face.

Sunlight: The sun can be viewed as medicine as its light converts the cholesterol on our skin into Vitamin D which helps in bone making. Vitamin D stimulates the absorption of calcium in the intestinal tract. Sunlight apparently provides immunity to cancer as it regulates the body's immune system. The absorption of the ultraviolet rays gives strength and vitality to the body. Sitting out in the sun among the flowers with the butterflies and birds flitting about in my garden felt soooo good!

Laughter raises the amount of natural killer cells in the blood and one of blood's jobs is to destroy tumor cells. I did not take Laughter 101 since my family is Laughter 101. We laugh a lot, especially when reminiscing.

Coconut Oil supposedly has anticancer properties. In days gone by, in my country, the only oil used was coconut. We were a lean population. Not many were diagnosed with cancer as they are today. We used it in our hair and rubbed it on our skin. It acted as a moisturizer. Not only was the coconut used for cooking, but also for baking. We made our own coconut oil then. I remember dropping a bottle of it when I was about 15 years old and my mother decided that I had to replace it. I trudged up to our garden which was about a mile away, gathered the coconuts, returned home and husked them. The next step was to break the shell, extract the kernel, and grate them. There were no blenders then. After the grating, water was added; the milk was extracted by squeezing with the hand. The milk was then put in a container for the fat to separate from the water. This was done by the fat floating to the top. The next step was to skim the fat off the top of the container with the final step being the boiling of the fat which turned into oil.

Salt: Some diets cut out salt completely, while others recommend sea salt. Salt is a vital mineral needed by the body as it carries nutrients to and from cells, among other functions. Yet, salt helps to retain fluid and can cause breast pain. According to one research, sea salt is moist and greyish in colour and recommends Celtic or Himalayan sea salt. I used the Celtic sea salt which was indeed moist and greyish in colour.

Chi Gong has been used to heal many diseases. It teaches you to use mind, body and spirit to unblock energy and create balance in the body. When the energy in the body is blocked, illnesses occur. Cancer is one of the illnesses which occur when the body's energy is blocked.

Yoga increases strength and our range of motion. It includes breathing and gentle stretches which has a calming influence on the body. The goal of yoga is a joining or union with God, the Eternal, the Divine, the Creator or whatever word with which you are comfortable. It strengthens the immune system and since cancer weakens the immune system, the use of yoga was added to my arsenal of non-conventional treatments to develop a strong healthy body and mind. Some of the poses showed me how stiff I was. Perhaps this stiffness resulted in the blockage of energy to different parts of the body.

Simple things like a beautiful sunset, soft ocean breezes, young animals or children at play and a sunrise create wonderment within the body in the form of peace, and drive away the cares of this life. I was fortunate to experience these where I live for I can see both sunset and sunrise, feel the soft ocean breezes, see young animals at play, as well as children, for my home is in the vicinity of a pre-school at which I volunteered my services.

There are more non-conventional weapons used in the war against cancer. This chapter listed those which I used.

There is so much information out there about food, that it can be confusing knowing what to do. Just when you think you have your perfect meal plan, something negative is being said about some of the foods. The importance of a good cancer diet is that it can help build the immune system and kill cancer cells. The immune system is the body's defense against diseases. It is made up of cells, tissues and organs which work to protect the body.

Know your individualized body and work with it. What is good for another may not be good for you and vice versa. Since you were individually made for your Creator's pleasure ("Know ye that the Lord he is God; it is he that hath made us, and not we ourselves..."(Psalms 100: 3, KJV)), He has a special interest in you. Trust Him.

CHAPTER 6

GOLDEN APPLES

A word fitly spoken is like apples of
gold in pictures of silver.
(Proverbs 25: 11, KJV)

1. Raw foods release more white blood cells.
2. Enzymes are needed by minerals and vitamins to reach the cells.
3. Raw foods build the immune system.
4. Antioxidants act as protectors for the body.
5. Selenium protects within the cells.
6. Vitamin E protects the outer cell membranes.
7. There are two kinds of Vitamin E: synthetic (dl-alpha-tocopherol) and natural (d-alpha-tocopherol). The natural stays longer in the body.
8. Sounds have the power to heal.
9. Laughter raises the amount of NK cells.
10. The immune system is the body's defense against disease.

TRUST AND FAITH

Put not your trust in princes, nor in the son
of man, in whom there is no help.
(Psalm 146: 3, KJV)

Trust and faith were the necessary tools I used to help
me with my choice of non-conventional treatment over
conventional - faith in the non-conventional treatment as
being the best way for me, and trust that it would work.
There was no looking back. There was no wondering if I
had made the right decision. I did not allow myself to doubt.

There are times when we are sure we have faith, but
when challenges arise, where faith is necessary, we find it
has disappeared. This was not one of those times. I took
the advice not to put my trust in princes or in man very
seriously for they could not help. I understood the spiritual

meaning behind not putting my trust in princes nor in the son of man in whom there is no help, as it applied to my diagnosis. What it meant to me was this: "Consider your fearfully and wonderfully-made body. Man did not make it. Put your trust in your Creator who made it."

My development of faith began with hope. A hope is more than a wish. A wish is just a passing thought without any action or roots, but a hope is more than a passing thought. It is positive, upbeat and alive. Because of this, you are waiting for your expectation to materialize. Hope is built on a firm foundation. It is unshaken. Do not allow your hope to waver.

No matter what happens, keep on hoping. Sometimes dark clouds and storms appear on the horizon, blocking our vision of what we are hoping for. These dark clouds and storms will pass. When they do, make sure your hope is still there for "hope deferred maketh the heart sick: but when the desire cometh, it is a tree of life" (Proverbs 13: 12, KJV). There is no time limit to a hope. Therefore we keep on hoping for we do not know when it will be fulfilled.

You have a part to play in the unfolding of your faith. That part is an active part. The development of faith is built one step at a time. We do not wake up one morning full of faith. It takes patience to develop faith, and when we have that faith, it also takes patience to wait for what we are faithful for to manifest itself. My development of faith came from remembering impossible situations over which I had no control that worked themselves out. I had nothing to do with the solutions. If those situations worked out then, I thought, surely other impossible situations like the healing of the cancer would work out too. The works required to keep faith alive is trust. Faith without trust is dead. To have trust is to have confidence, to believe, to know.

I avoided telling a lot of people about my diagnosis and choice of treatment, for I knew some would have tried to dissuade me. It would have made it harder to be free to exercise my will. Exercising my will is exercising my choice. In exercising my choice, I am breaking free from society and creating my own path. I am being myself for that is what I want to be; free to make my choice as to whether I should take conventional or non-conventional treatment.

Some people get upset when one goes against the established way of doing things. In trying to dissuade me from my choice, they would have placed a doubt in me as to whether my decision was the right one. This would have created a split personality - one who trusted and the other one who feared.

Sometimes it seems as though there are two of us: one who trusts and one who is afraid. The one who trusts knows that everything is fine. It lives outside of time. This is the one who knows that everything always works out because it looks beyond the appearance. It is also the one who knows that because its Creator lives outside of time, He could never come too late. It also knows that He works according to His timetable and not according to the timetable of the one who trusts. It also knows that worrying accomplishes nothing as it never helps and can never ever change any situation.

On the other hand, the one who fears is the one who worries, the one who walks by sight, the one who looks at appearances, the one who does not trust, the one who finds it hard to forgive, the one who chooses to believe that its

Creator does not care because it is not having its way, the one who is impatient, the one who wants everything now.

Faith is giving up what we can see, for what we cannot see. It is looking beyond the appearance. It is our faith that creates miracles. We were not given a spirit of fear, but of power and a sound mind. We are fearfully and wonderfully made, which means that we are to be held in high regard, to be in awe, amazement, respect and wonderment. We must remember this when our faith begins to waver. We owe it to our body to give it what it needs to restore its health.

A fearfully and wonderfully-made body does not mean that we should be afraid of it and do nothing to keep it wonderful. The word "fear" does not only mean to be afraid, but it also means *"to revere,"* which is to hold in great regard, to hold in awe. A fearfully and wonderfully-made body means that we are to hold it in awe, amazement, respect, wonderment. If we respect our body, we would take care of it.

We are empowered by not being given the spirit of fear but of power, for we are *"fearfully and wonderfully made."* We may know that we are empowered, but unless we use it by stepping out in faith, it is no good to us. If we do not use our power, it will be taken over by fear, just like a garden that is not tended is taken over by weeds. The more we use our power, the stronger we become and the more empowered we are.

Alongside faith is vision. Vision means to see the invisible which is not there, but it can also refer to one's eyesight. Imagination too is a part of vision as it is the ability to see mental images of something that exists in one's mind like your healing. Be a visionary. Look beyond the appearance of your state of health and see into your future healing now.

Faith and vision go hand in hand, as faith brings vision into being. The Apostle Paul says that we see through a glass darkly or, put another way, we see through an unclean glass and our vision is blocked, but if we were to clean the glass, we would see clearly. Applying faith to vision cleans the glass and causes the darkness to disappear. Faith helps us to look beyond the appearance of things. When our physical vision is failing, we wear glasses, contact lenses or have laser treatments to improve our eyesight. Faith improves our spiritual vision and helps us to see things more clearly.

"Where there is no vision, the people perish," (Proverbs 29: 18, KJV) but where there is vision the people flourish. To flourish is to thrive, to prosper. In the exercising of vision, we are stretching ourselves to look beyond the appearance, and asking how can this be improved? Beyond the appearance, there is always action. Visionaries like to be active and to flourish. When we envision, we choose and create a mental image of what we want. We want healing so we keep this vision alive, we give it power to materialize. Having vision causes us to endure. Life continually challenges us to greater growth, to greater expansion of ourselves, to stretch our limitless selves. Whatever you envision, take it to your Creator and he shall bring it to pass. "Commit thy way unto the Lord; trust also in him; and he shall bring it to pass" (Psalm 37: 5, KJV).

There is only one who heals. We have a healer who is no respecter of persons and on whom we can lean. Dr. Paracelsus, a Swiss German who lived from 1493 to 1541, understood that everything comes from nature, even sickness and healing. In his reference to cancer he states: "It should be forbidden and severely punished to remove cancer by cutting, burning, cautery and any fiendish tortures. It is from nature that diseases arise and from nature comes the cure."

Illness causes changes in us and is a great teacher. Since the body heals itself, there must be a healing code to be accessed. Being aware of our beliefs is a part of it. Do we believe that we can be healed? *"as thou hast believed, so be it done unto thee."* (Matthew 8:13, KJV) Our beliefs are powerful. The body responds to what the mind believes. My mind had to believe that healing comes from my Creator who made me (*"for I am the Lord that healeth thee"* (Exodus 15: 26, KJV)) and not from radiation or chemotherapy. Healing might have come through them as the instruments, but I did not accept these instruments because though they poison the cancer cells, they also destroy healthy cells and could cause damage to my organs like the liver, kidney and lungs of my wonderfully- made body.

The body is holy. It is the temple of your Creator. It knows what it needs to heal itself. Pay attention to it. Collect all the data you can. Research! Research! Research! Others have gone through the same thing before you. Take charge of your life. Do not hand it over to anyone. I knew I was not worrying or afraid about it because I slept well at nights. *"When thou liest down, thou shalt not be afraid; yea, thou shalt lie down and thy sleep shalt be sweet."* (Proverbs 3: 24, KJV)

We are afraid to go to sleep for different reasons. One of them is that we worry about our problems; another is that we are afraid of dying so that if we stay awake we know that we have not died. My dependency was on my Creator for a fearless and sweet sleep because I trusted Him. What He says, He does. Our Creator does not lie. We do. We make promises and break them.

Everything changes, but only our Creator is changeless. Seasons change into Spring, Summer, Autumn (Fall) and Winter in some parts of the world, and in others into rainy and dry seasons. We change from children into adults. Days change into nights. We live in a world of change. If our Creator were to change, could He be trusted? What about the promises He made? Could we take Him at His word? Would all things still be possible to those who believe? What if He were a respecter of persons?

These things will not happen for we know that He speaks Truth when He says, *"I change not."* In other words, I change not because I am Eternal – without beginning or end, everlasting, changeless. Everything is temporary, but only the Eternal is permanent, constant.

We can prove whether or not He is changeless, whether or not He means what He says. In fact, he does challenge us to prove Him, to test Him. King David, who wanted to know if he were on the right track, asked his Creator to examine him and prove him, to try his reins and his heart. We can prove our Creator by picking one of the promises He made to us and holding Him to it. After proving Him and armed with the knowledge that He is in indeed changeless and means what He says, nothing that happens should disturb or frighten us. I challenged my Creator to prove His own words to me: "I am the Lord that healeth thee." This challenge resulted in healing.

Be conscious of His presence and power at all times. Abraham was. He knew that his Creator was changeless. He trusted Him so much that he was willing to sacrifice his son to prove his faith in Him. Abraham was considered as His friend. His Creator spoke to him personally. He was with Abraham at all times, even though he was far from perfect and fearful at times.

The world is changing. Things are not what they used to be. That is true. This can be scary, but we can still live our lives with peace of mind knowing that our Creator is changeless. We know that His promises stand, including that of healing.

If our Creator has the power to make us peaceful by giving us the power of peace who or what can disturb or frighten us? If our Creator is for us, who or what can stand against us? If we prove that our Creator is changeless, and hold on to our proof, we will know that no one, no challenge, no sickness; no dis-ease can take our joy from us.

CHAPTER 7

GOLDEN APPLES

A word fitly spoken is like apples of
gold in pictures of silver.
(Proverbs 25: 11, KJV)

1. Everything comes from nature.
2. The body heals itself.
3. The body responds to what the mind believes.
4. The body is holy.
5. It is the temple of God.
6. Take charge of your life.
7. Imagination is a part of vision.
8. Faith and vision go hand in hand.
9. Faith improves our spiritual vision.
10. Imagination challenges the mind.
11. Imagination makes vision possible.
12. Life challenges us to greater expansion of ourselves.
13. Our thoughts are a necessary part in seeing.
14. Beyond the appearance there is always action.

CHAPTER 8

DEPENDENCY

Yet will they lean upon the Lord, and say, Is not the
Lord among us? None evil can come upon us.
(Micah 3: 11, KJV)

What is dependency?
How do we know we are in dependency?
On whom do we depend?
On whom should we depend?
When should we be dependent?

Dependency is leaning and expecting. This is what
children do. They depend on others, primarily parents, to
take care of them, to supply their needs, to right their wrongs
until they have matured to do those things themselves. This
is their way of life.

Dependency says that we do not quite measure up, therefore we look for someone to prop us up and hold us up. We depend on others when we feel weak, inadequate, frightened, deprived and/or unable to cope with life. Dependency creates a slave mentality on both the leaner and the leaned-on. It can become a habit if we keep on depending on others to provide our answers and support, instead of looking on the inside for the help needed. Sooner or later, this human dependency will create hostility.

We free ourselves from physical dependency by being fully aware of it (our dependencies). We are in dependency, when through fear or laziness, we hand our life over to someone else to make our decisions concerning our health.

On whom then should we depend? To depend on someone is to lean on them. Our dependency should be only on our Creator for His energy is always constant; it is always there; it can never be depleted. It is always flowing.

In our lifetime we will experience more than one challenge. One such challenge for me was the diagnosis of cancer. We seek explanations as to why sickness occurs. We look for rational explanations, but sometimes there are none. Our role is to accept and keep our faith in our Creator for He is always on our side.

His role is to stir up things, bring them together and deliver them to us, for He is a Creator of love. This love is not selfish for He causes the rain to fall both on the just and the unjust, meaning that He loves everyone – those of us who think we are righteous, and those of us who think we are not; those of us who believe in His existence, and those of us who do not; those of us who take conventional treatment, and those of us who do not.

Our minds are like gardens which need to be kept free of weeds so that healthy thoughts will prosper. Good and positive thoughts produce good fruits, whereas bad and negative thoughts produce bad fruits. My actions must reflect my thoughts. My thoughts should be that I am perfect and see myself doing everything I want to do energetically, easily and enthusiastically. I enjoy working in my flower garden. Visualizing myself doing this, gave me a new zest for living. There was no time to be sick. What I was developing was a health consciousness, not only for the duration of the dis-ease, but for the rest of my life. This did not mean that I was in denial.

Jesus said, *"As a man thinketh in his heart, so is he."* In other words, who and what I am is what I think about. If I think unhealthy thoughts, that is what I will be – unhealthy, even though I may be taking all the medication in the world. If I think healthy thoughts, that is what I will be – healthy. Healthy thoughts alone will not make me healthy. I can eat lots of junk food, sugar and salt and have healthy thoughts. Would this make me healthy? No. Healthy thoughts must be accompanied by action. This action is the doing of what is necessary to maintain a healthy body. I hold the key to my health and no one else. I have the power to alter my thoughts if they are going in the wrong direction. To do this, I have to be watchful over them.

My body was made to heal itself, hence *"my fearfully and wonderfully-made body,"* a body made from love, a body made with love. It is to be reverenced, wondered at and held in awe. It is made up of healing energy which is supposed to flow through freely, if healthy. Energy is power, like electricity is power.

Years ago, two friends were visiting. While watching a movie on television, the picture was unstable from time to time. Whenever I walked by, the picture became stable. Upon discovering this, I had to stand beside the set until the movie ended. Why am I telling you this? To show the power we have in our bodies without being aware of it.

Apparently, our bodies have about 50 trillion cells with 1.17 volts of electricity in each cell. Perhaps there are more since new discoveries are being made every day. With knowledge of this much power in my body, why should I not believe that it is capable of healing itself? If the energy/power in my body can stabilize a television set, what can it do to diseases within my body? Our body is made up of different sizes and structure of cells, tissues and organs. An organ is a part of the body which performs a special work. For example, the stomach is an organ of digestion, the eye is the organ of sight, the tongue is the organ of speech. Some organs may have more than one function. Our body consumes fuel, stores up energy and produces movement. It has life and attends to its own needs. It repairs itself. It is capable of growth and reproduction. It regulates its own body temperature and removes its own waste. This is our fearfully and wonderfully-made body!

Sometime ago, I visited a property in the *"bush"* which had a river running through it. The water was so clear that I could see the white sand at its bottom. Lower down, there was a blockage caused by leaves and pieces of twigs. These prevented the free flow of water, which resulted in stagnation. Unless the blockage was removed, parts of the river would eventually dry up. However, with the removal of the blockage, the river would flow freely again. So it is with our body. Care must be taken of all parts of the body for it to function properly. When we have blockages, if they are not removed for our energy to flow freely, we become sick and disease-ridden.

Our *"fearfully and wonderfully-made body"* was also made to heal itself with the supply of energy points located throughout the body. The hands are one of the instruments used for unblocking the stagnation of energy from any area of the body, thus resulting in healing by the free flow of energy to that area.

When any part of our body is hurt and we rub our hands together until they are warm and either cover the part and/or massage the area, healing takes place. Try it. Knowing this, I rubbed my hands together, creating some warmth, and placed them on the affected breast, from time to time.

Jesus knew that the body was made to heal itself, therefore when he healed someone by touch, he would have unblocked the energy in that area, causing it to flow freely once more. He introduced us to our Creator, our Healer, the one who stirs up things, brings them together, and then delivers them to us, not as a man, but as Spirit. *"God is a Spirit: and they that worship him must worship him in spirit and in truth"* (John 4: 24, KJV). Healing requires faith, one that does not waver. A wavering faith is unprofitable.

CHAPTER 8

GOLDEN APPLES

A word fitly spoken is like apples of
gold in pictures of silver.
(Proverbs 25: 11, KJV)

1. Dependency is leaning and expecting.
2. Dependency creates a slave mentality.
3. Depend only on your Creator.
4. Our minds are like gardens which need to be kept free of weeds so healthy thoughts will prosper.
5. You hold the key to your health and no one else.
6. Your body was made to heal itself.
7. Energy is power.
8. Healing requires faith.
9. A wavering faith is unprofitable.

THE WAIT

"Wait for the Lord and he will deliver you."
(Proverbs 20: 22, NIV)

Though we may or may not understand why we are in a challenge, waiting for it to end gets to us. We have done all we can to help the situation and have turned it over to our Creator for whom nothing is impossible; "But why is the wait taking so long?" we ask.

Waiting is a part of life. It builds patience. It builds character. It builds trust. Look beyond the appearance that you are alone while you wait, for you are never alone. How can you be alone when you are breathing in and out? The breath that you are breathing in and out is your Creator's breath. It was breathed into you at your creation. "And the Lord God formed man of the dust of the ground, and breathed into his nostrils the breath of life; and man became a living soul" (Genesis 2: 7, KJV). You are the body. He is the breath. Without His breath the body has no life. The words *"I will never leave you nor forsake you"* are Truth for as long as you are breathing, He has not left you nor forsaken you.

What we do while we wait can make a difference to shorten the time. We need a distraction while we wait, for our mind will keep rehashing the challenge over and over, making it bigger than it already is. Removing ourselves from the center of attention and showing love towards others by helping and serving wherever we can, will shorten the wait. When we make a work out of serving and putting our heart into it, time goes quickly. My distraction was my garden and volunteer work at a pre-school.

Time is like a two-sided coin. It is both the enemy and the friend of man. It is the enemy because of the waiting period it involves. When we want something, we want it now not later, not in some distant future, but today, now, immediately! Waiting on time creates anxieties, frustrations, fears, illnesses, sadness. It moves ever so slowly, especially if we cannot see an end in sight to the challenge. It is our nature to worry and be anxious *"for we see through a glass darkly."* Everything looks bleak.

Yet it is the slowness of time which heals and teaches. This makes it the friend of man. It gives us the opportunity to make a fresh start. It is necessary for our unfoldment, for the development of our character, for the building of our faith. It is the key which releases anxieties, frustrations, fears, illnesses and sadness. This we realize in hindsight.

The most important challenge is to be positive while we wait. A useful tool while we wait is meditation. Meditation is deep reflection, a reflection on the spiritual, the Creator within. It is a retreat, a revelation into our own mind. It is making contact with the One Great Mind, the only mind which exists. What better way to face the day than with morning meditation to help one cope with the daily stress of life!

In meditation, one's life is changed by the acquiring of spiritual development. One finds peace of mind, comfort and reassurance within. It is a place where outside forces cannot enter. It changes our perspective, giving us a new sense of identity, awareness of strengths and resources, increased feelings of personal rights, culminating in a zest for life.

Meditation is not only a means of gaining peace, raising our energy levels or providing healing. In meditation the ego is deposed. The focus is no longer on the self without, but on the self within. In meditation, the "what" surfaces. The world around is closed out. It is forgotten as one is transported into another world.

When one has recognition of one's Higher Self that one is the vessel in whom his/her Creator lives, one can live life fully, knowing the outcome. Communion with our Creator gives us the peace of mind we need in our life and affairs. It opens up awareness, pulling us away from the ego as we ascend to a higher level of consciousness.

Another useful tool while we wait is prayer. Prayer is an admission that no matter how big we think we are, there is someone or something bigger. No matter how much in control we think we are, there is One with even greater control. It is a unification of God and man, a union of you and your Creator. It is an acknowledgment that there is a solution for whatever we are praying about. Prayer links our mind to God's Mind. When we pray, we are in a higher level of consciousness.

Jesus said that "Men ought always to pray..." and he did teach us how to pray. One such instruction is "When you pray, enter into your closet and when you have shut the door, pray to your Father which is in secret and your Father who sees in secret shall reward you openly." In other words when we pray, enter into the closet of our minds and shut everything out.

Waiting for what we think is a long time creates doubt, but it is by waiting that we create the faith necessary for waiting. Be courageous. Stop worrying. He has not forgotten you. Your time has not yet come. He is still preparing you to receive all that He has for you. As the Master Potter, He is molding and shaping you into the vessel He needs for His work. You are in the best possible hands. The Master Potter would never drop you. He will never forget you in the kiln. "Can a woman forget her nursing child, or show no compassion for the child of her womb? Even these may forget, yet I will not forget you" (Isaiah 49: 15, NRSV). Healing requires faith, one that does not waver. A wavering faith is unprofitable. Hang in there!

CHAPTER 9

GOLDEN APPLES

A word fitly spoken is like apples of
gold in pictures of silver.
(Proverbs 25: 11, KJV)

1. We need a distraction while we wait.
2. Time is like a two-sided coin – the enemy of man and the friend of man.
3. Waiting on time creates anxieties, frustrations, fears, illnesses and sadness.
4. It is our nature to worry and be anxious "for we see through a glass darkly."
5. Be positive while you wait.
6. A useful tool while you wait is meditation.
7. Prayer is a unification of God and man.
8. Waiting is a part of life.
9. It builds patience, character and trust.
10. It is by waiting that we create the faith necessary for waiting.

CHAPTER 10

DEATH

What man is he that liveth, and shall not see death?
(Psalms 89: 48, KJV)

When someone heard that I was not going the conventional route of radiation and/or chemotherapy, the remark was *"Does she want to die?"* Radiation/chemotherapy would not have saved my life. If it were my belief that they would, I would have taken that route.

So many have used these conventional treatments and have died. We all have to die sooner or later, though why not go later than sooner? I had no intention of dying then. I enjoyed life. There were things I had yet to accomplish like learning how to play the violin to accompany the children at Philma's Early Childhood Center where I volunteered. The principal is an accomplished violin, clarinet, piano and cello player. Volunteering at the Center opened the door for me to learn whatever instruments I chose.

When I met with the oncologist and he explained the necessity for radiation, I replied "People take radiation and chemotherapy and they die, they don't take it and they die." His response was, "We all die," to which I said: "That's my point." My point was radiation/chemotherapy would not save my life and knowing that, why go through the side effects?

Death is a cessation of life as we know it. It is the fulfillment of our life's purpose on earth. Why this fear of death, anyway? Is it because we do not know what is beyond it? The concept of heaven painted as a wonderful picture of drinking milk and honey and staring into our Creator's face (or perhaps that has since changed) should make us long for it in our hurry to get there. Nevertheless, we fear death and very seldom talk about it, yet that is the only known way to enter the concept of heaven, if it is a part of your belief.

Fear of death prevents us from living fully. As we grow older, death gets closer. We must understand what death means to us and deal with it. Death to me was not an end to life, but a beginning of another. I did not want to die, so I did everything in my power to stay alive. My not wanting to die had nothing to do with fear. There were many things I still had to accomplish, one of which was to make a chemical-free vegetable garden to feed myself. A chemical-free garden is referred to as an organic garden.

Our gardens were fertilized with animal manure. These animals ate grass for their food. Today we have grass-fed meat, grass-fed butter, grass-fed this, grass-fed that, free-range chicken, free-range eggs. The word free-range was not known either. The way of growing organically today, was the way we grew our food and raised our animals way back then. The words organic and free-range were known, but not in the context with the growing of food or the rearing of animals or chickens.

One does not need cancer to die. People die without having an illness. If we are to believe that there is an appointed time, then when that time comes, whether ill or not, do we have a choice? It helps us accept death if we make it a part of life, for it is. What dies? the essence of the person, or the body which houses the essence? Death is with us at all times, from the moment we enter this world to the time we leave it, or put another way, from the time of our creation to the time we expire. This can happen at any time.

Though I said I did not want to die, what if I knew I had a certain number of months or years to live? How would I spend it? Would the material things, the fussing and fighting matter anymore? How important would be the competition and the comparison? Self-examination would seem to be the most important thing to do in preparation for the ending of this life as I know it. What about you? What would you do?

My 85-year old sister knew the secret to life and death, for before her stroke she was ready to leave this world as she knew it. She had no near-death experiences that we knew of. She was not ill. What was it that she knew that we, her family, did not know? My sister did not believe in reincarnation, which is a concept that we die and come back as somebody else but maintain the essence. She never mentioned why she wanted to go, or where she was going. She was unafraid of death. She accepted the life and death cycle. Six months after having the stroke she got her wish. Though we missed her, we did not grieve. We knew it was what she wanted. Her acceptance of death as being inevitable and meeting it head-on in a calm, accepting way was a great lesson to the family.

The fear of death is understandable because we do not know what it is. What we know is that everyone dies. We do not know where we go. Perhaps my sister knew what the Apostle Paul did. Whatever happens after death, the Apostle Paul looked forward to it. In speaking to the Corinthians, he removes this fear for us by saying if he had a choice, he would rather be with the Lord. *"We are confident, I say, and willing rather to be absent from the body, and to be present with the Lord."* (11 Corinthians 5: 8, KJV)

Paul was torn between a desire to depart to be with Christ and a desire to abide in the flesh. Though he showed that the better of the two desires was to be with Christ, he nevertheless recognized that he had to be in the flesh because he was needed on earth to do the job for which he was created. He had to complete his job until his appointed time came for him to be with the Lord.

To him it was not an end, but a beginning. It was a different way of life. Death also shows how fearfully and wonderfully made our body is for everything ceases, the body shuts itself off. This is a miracle. Fear of death stops us from living joyfully. In some cases, death could be the perfect healing tool. My sister, a stroke patient, died in six months, while some live for years bedridden. Death was the perfect healing tool for her.

My not taking radiation/chemotherapy has nothing to do with my wanting to die, for whether or not I take it,

I have to wait until my appointed time. *"Is there not an appointed time to man upon earth?"* (Job 7: 1, KJV) "Seeing his days are determined, the number of his months are with thee, thou hast appointed his bounds that he cannot pass" (Job 14: 5, KJV). So what if I die? My belief is that my appointed time will have come. Can I do anything about it? No.

CHAPTER 10

GOLDEN APPLES

A word fitly spoken is like apples of
gold in pictures of silver.
(Proverbs 25: 11, KJV)

1. Everyone dies.
2. Our days are numbered.
3. Death is the fulfillment of our life's purpose on earth.
4. Fear of death prevents us from living fully.

THE SURGERY

Choose this day whom you will serve.
(Joshua 24: 15, NRSV)

In refusing to do a mastectomy, I chose to have a lumpectomy instead. My nephew, Garth, drove me to the hospital on the morning of the surgery. After it was over, I was wheeled into the Women's Ward where I spent a night and part of the following day, hooked up on IV's – those tubes that drip, drip, drip whatever it is into the veins. Hospital food generally has a bad name but I enjoyed it. Perhaps I was hungry for when one is hungry, anything tastes good.

A lumpectomy removes the least amount of breast tissue. In this procedure, the cancer and a small portion or margin of the surrounding tissue is removed. This is the least invasive breast cancer surgery. This operation leaves the breast smaller, different in shape and a bit firmer. The removed breast tissue was sent to the pathologist – a physician - who looked at the edges for cancer cells. After the first biopsy to determine the diagnosis of cancer, a second biopsy - the Sentinel Lymph Node Biopsy - was done to find out the stage of the cancer and to estimate the risk of whether tumor cells had developed the ability to spread to other parts of the body.

A Sentinel Lymph Node is the first lymph node to which cancer cells are likely to spread from a tumor. In preparation for my Sentinel Lymph Node Biopsy, an overnight fast, a chest x-ray, an ECG and blood tests and the signing of a consent form were done. After being put to sleep, a blue dye was injected near the tumor to locate the sentinel lymph node and/or other nodes stained with the blue dye. Once the sentinel lymph node is located, a small incision was made and the nodes removed.

Lymph nodes are part of our lymphatic system and are located in the neck, underarms, chest, abdomen and groin. These nodes are connected to one another by lymph vessels. The lymph comes from a fluid leaked out of small blood vessels which travels through the lymph vessels into the lymph nodes. Lymph nodes are part of our immune system. The immune system made up of cells, tissues and organs is the body's defense against infections. Since lymph nodes are a part of the immune system, a lymph node biopsy disrupts the flow of lymph to the immune system. In cutting the nodes, the normal flow of lymph through the affected area is disrupted. This disruption created a buildup of lymph fluid, swelling and pain. The area became thickened and hard. Hopefully, with time, this will return to normal.

Like everything else, sentinel lymph node biopsy has its good and bad. It can give a false negative result that cancer cells are not present when they are. On the plus side, it is used to help stage breast cancer.

Some doctors are against the removal of lymph nodes (even though the removal and analysis are part of how a surgeon determines how far the cancer has spread and are used to make treatment decisions) because of swelling and pain in the arm which does not always go away. The lymph nodes are part of the body's immune system and help the body fight cancer.

Visits were made to the local clinic for the dressing of the wound, after which I was referred to the Oncology Department. After a lumpectomy, radiation is the prescribed therapy to rid the body of any remaining cancer cells where the tumor was located. The Oncologist did suggest the radiation therapy but I refused. Radiation not only destroys cancer cells, but also burns and damages the cells, tissues and organs that are healthy.

Hormone Replacement Therapy in the form of Anastrozole or Arimidex was then recommended to me as it is supposed to block the formation of new blood vessels by tumors. The tumors rely on blood vessels for the oxygen and nutrients in order to survive. The drug can block the protein that helps the formation of blood vessels in the tumor.

Tamoxifen is the drug most often used as it locks estrogen out of breast cancer cells to prevent them from growing. Cruciferous vegetables like cabbage, broccoli, kale, Brussels sprouts and turnips contain indole-3-carbinol which decreases the ability of estrogen from binding to breast tissue. A low-fat diet also helps to relieve breast pain by reducing estrogen levels, as does fiber which helps estrogen from over-stimulating breast tissue. Iodine can also be used to relieve breast pain.

Broccoli, Brussels sprouts and cauliflower are not common in my part of the world, nor are the berries, though they are imported as "fresh" or frozen. By the time the fresh ones arrive, how fresh are they? I used both "fresh" and frozen.

I visited a cancer center for a follow-up and Tamoxifen *20mg once a day or Arimidex 1mg for five years* was recommended, but I discovered the side effects could result in uterine cancer. I refused to take either one of them for their negative side effects outweighed their good. Why trade one cancer for another? It made no sense to me, for whatever I would take for uterine cancer caused by side effects, could also result in another type of cancer. It would be like being on a merry-go-round.

CHAPTER 11

GOLDEN APPLES

A word fitly spoken is like apples of
gold in pictures of silver.
(Proverbs 25: 11, KJV)

1. A lumpectomy removes the least amount of breast tissue.
2. It is the least invasive breast cancer surgery.
3. Iodine can be used to relieve breast pain.
4. Lymph nodes are part of our lymphatic system connected to one another by lymph vessels.
5. They are part of our immune system.
6. Tamoxifen is the drug most often used in the treatment of cancer.
7. Cabbage, broccoli, kale, Brussels sprouts and turnips contain indole-3-carbinol which decreases the ability of estrogen from binding to breast tissue.

SUMMING UP

> The eternal God is thy refuge, and underneath are the
> everlasting arms: and he shall thrust out the enemy
> from before thee; and shall say, Destroy them.
> (Deuteronomy 33: 27, KJV)

The enemy is whatever takes our joy from us. When things go wrong, we wonder why and expect them to be fixed immediately. Seldom do we see them as things over which we are to be joyful. Instead, they are seen as things which have come to try us again and again and again! They are painful and cause suffering. They try our patience. They try our faith. They are exhausting.

Yet, according to the Apostle Peter, we are not to think it strange when things go wrong. Instead we are to rejoice in them. The Apostle James refers to them as trials which come upon us to test our faith.

Life requires of us that we live it to its fullest. The fiery trials which are trying us are challenging us to climb higher, to go in a new direction in order to partake of something of value because we can rise to the occasion. *"His divine power has given us everything needed for life and godliness."* To live this life and to acquire this godliness requires faith for *"human beings are born to trouble just as sparks fly upwards."* It is this trouble which builds our faith and helps us develop godly traits.

For the development of this faith, one requires endurance. Endurance must be fueled by passion. Without it endurance will not last. How does passion fuel endurance? It expresses an emotion of great depth, of great feeling. It is a very strong conviction of a right to your need, whether it be the need to right the wrong, the need to see the end of your trial, the need for peace of mind, the need to live life to its fullest, the need to develop godly traits or whatever need we think of as our entitlement, like the need for healing.

This conviction causes us to endure. We have gone beyond the known boundaries, beyond the surface into the vast realm of the unknown. When we are passionate about something, it is to know that our belief in whatever it is, is the one and only truth, contrary to all appearances.

How I Dealt with Cancer in a Non-Conventional Way encourages you to keep on enduring, to keep on persevering, to keep on climbing, to keep on looking beyond the appearance when things go wrong "so that you may be mature and complete, lacking in nothing." We take so much for granted until something happens for us to take stock. We each have various stages of challenges. My bout with cancer could have been a *"dark night of the soul"*, but I chose not to make it so. It could have been a death sentence, but again I chose not to make it so.

"The Dark Night of the Soul" was a classic piece of work written in the 16th century by Saint John of the Cross. His writing was about the personal spiritual journey. Since then, the deep trials we go through that almost break us so that we say "My God, My God why have you forsaken me?" have been termed *"the dark night of the soul."*

Everyone has a dark night of the soul. If you haven't, prepare yourself. It is coming! When we are in the dark night of the soul, our thoughts are not rational. This irrationality goes on and on, sometimes to the point of despair. When we despair, what we are saying is there is no hope. In thinking like that, our thought is that our Creator is dead, and there is no one to get us out of the hole we are in or that He has abandoned us. Our thoughts will go in this direction because the situation we are in is unbearable and we want out now!

It is said that the treatment of heat is absolutely critical to bring out the best in steel; therefore, the best steel must go through the fire. For you to transform into the best steel, you too must go through the fire. If you are experiencing "the dark night of the soul", remember why you are doing so. It is to "add to your faith virtue; and to virtue knowledge; and to knowledge temperance; and to temperance patience and to patience godliness; and to godliness brotherly kindness; and to brotherly kindness charity" (11 Peter 1:5-7, KJV).

Our *dark night of the soul* should make us pay attention to everything that is taking place within it, for the possibility exists that there is something that can be shared with others to benefit them. Dark nights of the soul are never for us alone, but for others as well. "Wherefore lift up the hands which hang down, and the feeble knees; and make straight paths for your feet…" (Hebrews 12: 12-13, KJV). In other words, stop moaning and groaning, be active, do something. Take action!

My weight was down by 20lbs, my clothes and shoes were much too big and I looked and still do look like a scarecrow. I lost so much weight then, that it was uncomfortable sitting on wooden chairs. My sitting bones were devoid of fat but I feel great now as I eat fruits, vegetables, fish (steamed but fried now and then), take a few vitamins like selenium, Vitamin E, COQ10, Evening Primrose Oil, B12, Omega 3 Flaxseed Oil and a multivitamin. I also exercise, do chi gong, yoga, sit in the sun doing crossword puzzles and/or read and listen to music. The changing of my lifestyle is not a knee-jerk change, but is to be continued for the rest of my life. The buying of fish is challenging. I remember once buying salmon steaks and leaving it in water. When I returned, the steaks were a pale grey and the water colored. The fish was dyed. This was my first introduction to farm-raised fish.

When I lost weight from my change of diet, I was troubled and confused, for when I looked in the mirror, the person looking back at me was not me. I looked different. The confusion came about because who I thought I was did not match what I saw on the outside. The inside did not match the outside. The image I was comfortable with all my life had changed. It seemed as though the dis-ease had created two different persons. I avoided looking in the mirror, for I did not want to see this other person. I had to change my thoughts to accept this new person. I wondered if others felt my strangeness. It took me a long, long time to merge both parts of me – the inner and the outer.

Was I transforming? Was I becoming a new person? Was I shedding who I thought I was to become who I could be? Was that why I felt so uncomfortable? Was it time for me to leave the old behind and embrace the new? When the body is not at ease, all its parts are affected spiritually, mentally, physically and emotionally. Apparently, the time had come to release the old me and create a new me. We cannot be the same person after a challenge. Life requires of us that we transform. Without transformation we are boring.

The process of transformation can be likened to that of a caterpillar which changes into a butterfly. The change from the caterpillar into the butterfly is symbolic of rebirth after death, as the caterpillar is seen as being dead before the butterfly can emerge. Experiencing a life-threatening dis-ease like cancer, where the very mention of the word conjures up death, is like a transformation from a caterpillar into a beautiful butterfly. We become different people for we change and turn away from our former way of life. We eat differently; we exercise and do whatever it takes to keep the body healthy. The caterpillar cannot fly, but by changing into a butterfly it is able to fly wherever it chooses. Like the butterfly, we do things we never knew we could have done before.

My body, now being tired of raw food, enjoys stir-fry for lunch. I enjoy preparing this since I grow most of the produce like patchoi, tomatoes, sweet peppers, flavor peppers, melongene (eggplant or aubergine depending on your location) peas, ochroes (okra), cabbage, turmeric and herbs like celery, marjoram, mint, basil, garlic, chives, tarragon.

This is the preparation for the stir-fry. The produce is cut up into small pieces. Prepare your vegetables when you are ready to make the stir-fry to avoid destroying some of the vitamins. The base consists of patchoi (pak choi or Bok choy), onions, garlic and tomatoes. Patchoi, pak choi or Bok choy is a leafy green vegetable which is easy to grow and takes about a month to reap. It is rich in Vitamin C, fiber and folic acid. The plant with green stem is known as patchoi or pak choi; the plant with the white stem is known as Bok choy. The one I use has a white stem and should be called Bok choy, but whether green stem or white stem, it serves the same purpose.

The base is sautéed in coconut oil, olive oil or sesame oil to which is added turmeric powder and geera (cumin). In my part of the world, geera is another name for cumin. Any other vegetables can be added with some hot pepper to spice it up. Occasionally, I add some almond or Brazilian nuts, pumpkin seeds, sunflower seeds. Sometimes I accompany it with quinoa, couscous, beans or fish. The brown quinoa is delicious. My family loves visiting at lunch time.

My breakfast now consists of a smoothie. Each day is different, with the base being old-fashioned oats which is digested more slowly than quick-cooking oats, carrots, flaxseeds, cinnamon, almond or hemp milk and honey. Honey is a natural sweetener with proteins, minerals and vitamins. To this can be added strawberry and a banana or raspberries, papaw, blueberries, mangoes and/or nuts or whatever your imagination concocts. It is all up to you. I make it thick and freeze some of it for a pretend ice cream. It is delicious.   I do not use cold cuts or soft drinks. I snack on almonds, walnuts, pumpkin seeds, sunflower seeds and dark chocolate with a content of 70% cocoa. It is bitter but nice-tasting.

I rub myself with warmed sesame oil before taking a bath as heat helps in the absorption of the oil and opens up blood vessels. I discovered that when purchasing sesame oil one has to be careful, for some brands are mixed with other oils and therefore are not 100 percent pure sesame oil. Remember our skin is very sensitive because of nerve receptors. When we are touched, these receptors in the skin are activated. The fingertips have a large concentration of nerve receptors and a high degree of sensitivity. Thus, when we touch ourselves or someone else, we can send healing chemicals into the bloodstream as the skin is the richest source of hormones and immune cells.

There is power in our fingertips. We touch with our fingers which are part of our hands. *You open your hand, satisfying the desire of every living thing*" (Psalms 145:16, NRSV). Our Creator sets us the example of opening up His hands to satisfy our desires. When we close our hands, our fingertips are bent inwards and nothing can enter or leave. By opening our hands, our fingertips are free for touching to aid in our desire for healing.

I avoided dairy products as much as possible and used and still use almond milk (beverage). I was warned to look for the word "Carrageenan" in the ingredients. It is a food additive made from red seaweed used as a thickening agent and is supposedly non-digestible.

As with everything else, some researchers say it is safe, while others say it is not. The rule I follow is "When in doubt, don't." The word is omitted on some almond milk (beverage) boxes, while others specifically say "No Carrageenan." I have also seen it listed on some ice cream brands.

CHAPTER 12

GOLDEN APPLES

A word fitly spoken is like apples of
gold in pictures of silver.
(Proverbs 25: 11, KJV)

1. Life requires of us that we live it to its fullest.
2. For the development of faith, one requires endurance.
3. Everyone has a dark night of the soul.
4. There is power in our fingertips.

CHAPTER 13

THE STAGES

Someone asked me what "Stage" of cancer I was in. I was unaware that there were stages until asked the question. Knowing the Stage was not important to me for it would have meant acceptance of what I considered to be an unwanted, unwelcomed and uninvited thing. My acceptance would have given it life.

Knowing what Stage I was in would have caused me to think about the next "Stage" and the next and the next. My mind would not have been at rest, as it would have been worrying about the next Stage. Why create unnecessary anxiety? My preoccupation was about putting my body at ease through the healing of the dis-ease instead of worrying about the next Stage which would have been putting my mind into the future and not into the now. In this case, ignorance was bliss.

However, in researching the stages, I discovered that there are five. Stage 0 is the first and is the most treatable. In this stage, abnormal cells are detected within the top layer of cells in a localized area. When these abnormal cells clump together and penetrate under the top layer, this is referred to as Stage 1. Generally, when a small tumor is formed from the cancerous cells which have not spread to other parts of the body, this is referred to as Stage 11. Stage 111 is the spreading of the tumor into lymph nodes and surrounding tissues as it grows and Stage IV, the final stage, occurs when the cancer cells are no longer localized, but spread to another part or parts of the body.

The mention of the word "cancer" drives fear into our hearts. Our focus should not be dwelling on the stage, but on the determination to right the body. Find out why the immune system is not doing its job. Fix it and get the cancer out. The emphasis should be on the cancer and not on the stage. Why is the stage of importance when the treatment is the same for all? Knowledge of the stage can prevent healing, for if I am told I am in Stage IV which is known as the final stage, why would I bother to fight it? Aren't we told that this is the stage when death is inevitable? My thinking would be I am dying anyway. Whatever hope I might have had is soon dashed.

One of the first things we do when we greet each other is to enquire after one's health. We make a habit out of asking "How are you?" Our automatic response is "I am fine, I am okay." The one being asked the question knows that this exchange which is taking place is being done out of customary habit which is two parts of a greeting and nothing more.

However, if we have been diagnosed with cancer and are being greeted by someone who may be aware of it or not, when asked the question, "How are you?" answer truthfully, instead of saying, "I am okay, everything's fine." You are not okay and you are not fine. Your answering truthfully to some unaware of your diagnosis may create an awkward moment for we still have this fear of the <u>word</u> "cancer." Be prepared for that and put them at ease by telling them how you are handling it. Engage them in a discussion about it. You may be helping them to remove their fear of the dis-ease.

Whatever stage of the dis-ease one is in, it is traumatic. People genuinely want to help, for no one is exempt from cancer. The probability is there for all of us since it is said that we all have these cells within us. When we do not answer correctly, we could be denying help from our Creator for He works through us and could be sending you a message of hope in the form of something to use or someone to see.

We cannot expect help from others if we hide ourselves. There is nothing shameful about being diagnosed with cancer. We all have cells, some of which can become cancerous. Some of us are diagnosed with cancer, and others are not. For those diagnosed with it, their body is not at ease and those not diagnosed with it, their body is at ease. Our job then is to put the body at ease. That's all it is. There is nothing shameful about that. On the other hand, could it be that we think something is wrong with us, some failing we have why we are the ones with the dis-ease, and not those from whom we are hiding? As such we hide our imperfectness from their perfectness. Could that be it?

Sometimes we do not want others to know for fear of being pitied. There is that word again – fear. Pity is nothing but love. It is something we feel when others are suffering. It comes from the heart which is the seat of love and is one of the choicest gifts of our Creator. The heart feels while the head reasons. Our reasoning can be influenced by our thoughts, while the heart has no reasoning to do. It just feels; it just knows.

- Love is doing.
- Love is thoughtful.
- Love is patient.
- Love is caring.
- Love is trustworthy.
- Love inspires confidence.
- Love encourages.
- Love is fearless.
- Love is bold.
- Love is compassion.
- Love is our Creator.

Some of us are private and do not share our challenges, either because we do not want to burden anyone or we feel exposed, unprotected and/or vulnerable. But the diagnosis of cancer has created its own industry of cancer coaching. Those who have gone through the trauma of this dis-ease of the body are mentoring others. This is good, for the best coach is the one who deeply feels what you are going through; the one who can communicate with you at your level. This will remove the frustration of opening up to someone who has no idea what you are talking about or how to comfort. I did not have a cancer coach. I was not aware of any at that time.

The stages seem to be of importance to some. To my way of thinking, focus should not be placed on the stage or type, but on the cancer itself. That is the common threat to the body. From my understanding the treatment for all stages is the same used in conventional treatment – radiation, chemotherapy, hormone replacement therapy and in the case of non-conventional treatment – diet, exercise, a radical change in lifestyle.

A question I am asked is, "Are you in remission?" What is remission? The dictionary's explanation is *a lessening of a disease or illness.* When someone is in remission, is he/she healed? Remission of cancer to my way of thinking is that it has not left the body, but is hiding somewhere only to resurface years later.

What is interesting about the diagnosis is this, when in my thirties, I had a thermography test done. In this procedure, the breast is not touched as in mammography where it is compressed. I was left alone for about fifteen minutes in a very cold room after disrobing the top part for my body to reach the temperature of the room. When it did, I was placed in front of an infrared imaging camera where the top part of my body was imaged. At that time I was advised to pay attention to the left breast, the same one which later developed an abnormality of cells.

What did pay attention mean? Watch what you eat? Exercise? Reduce stress levels? Perhaps if I knew then, what I know now, how to take care of my body, there would have been no diagnosis. But, then, there would have been nothing to share with you.

The cancer served its purpose as a signal, a warning that all was not well with my body and that it required maintenance. It also served another purpose in introducing me to my fearfully and wonderfully-made body. It is well with my body for I now take care of it. I now maintain it. Emphasis is placed on the "now" for we tend to put off things into the future, without realizing that the future is "now". It also helped with my unfurling.

My family, friends and doctor respected my decision about not taking chemotherapy or radiation or hormone replacement therapy and did not try to change my mind. However, some, including family members, knowing that I did not have a mastectomy or took the conventional route of radiation, chemotherapy or hormone replacement therapy, thought I was misdiagnosed. If it were a misdiagnosis, do I have any regrets? No. Whether or not it was a misdiagnosis, knowledge was gained from it: Knowledge of how I am wonderfully made; knowledge which I did not have before and knowledge to share with you and the creation of a new me. Such knowledge is priceless!

CHAPTER 13

GOLDEN APPLES

A word fitly spoken is like apples of
gold in pictures of silver.
(Proverbs 25: 11, KJV)

1. Tumors rely on blood vessels for oxygen and nutrients in order to survive.
2. Vegetables like cabbage, broccoli, kale, Brussels sprouts and turnips can decrease estrogen from binding to breast tissue.
3. There are five stages of cancer: Stage 0 has abnormal cells within the top layer of cells in a localized area; in Stage I, the abnormal cells clump together and penetrate under the top layer; in Stage II, a small tumor is formed from the cancerous cells which have not spread to other parts of the body; in Stage III, the tumor spreads into lymph nodes and surrounding tissues as it grows and in Stage IV, the cancer cells are no longer localized, but have spread to another part or parts of the body.

BE THANKFUL

Giving thanks always for all things unto God and
the Father in the name of our Lord Jesus Christ.
(Ephesians 3: 20, KJV)

The Apostle Paul wrote letters to the Ephesians. In one of
them he mentioned the giving of thanks always for all things
unto our Creator. This message was not for the Ephesians
only, but for all of us today and forever. He did not mention
what specific things to give thanks for. He did not separate
the good from the bad, but put them together as all things.
In other words, whatever situation we are in, good or bad,
give thanks.

All things are considered to be good depending on how
we view them. If we consider "all things" as challenges
and hand them over to the Creator who created us, we

will emerge victorious. "Behold I am the Lord, the God of all flesh: is there any thing too hard for me (Jeremiah 32: 27, KJV)?" One of my friends, on the day he was declared cancer-free; decided to go for a bicycle ride in celebration. He was hit by a car. While lying in the road, he gave thanks. He mentioned that two verses came to him:

1. "And we know that all things work together for good to them that love God, to them who are the called according to his purpose." (Romans 8: 28, KJV) and

2. "Giving thanks always for all things unto God and the Father in the names of our Lord Jesus Christ" (Ephesians 3: 20, KJV).

He wondered what good would have come from the accident. The good resulted in forgiveness and a new friendship formed between his family and the family of the one who caused the accident.

If everything in our lives went smoothly, we would be bored. We need challenges to do some pearling. When a parasite, a piece of shell, or grain of sand, or a bit of stray food accidentally gets in between one of the two shells of an oyster, it goes pearling. Since it cannot expel the irritant, the oyster eases itself by covering the irritant with layers of nacre, the same mineral substance that made its shell. The irritant covered with layers and layers of this silky crystalline substance has now become a pearl.

Comparison can be drawn between us and the oyster. Since the oyster cannot eject the irritator, it goes a-pearling. It uses part of itself to cover the irritator for relief and this action creates something beautiful from which we benefit. We adorn ourselves with pearls and benefit financially. We should thank the oyster for its wisdom in handling the irritator.

When we have challenges from which we cannot escape, we need to go a-pearling. The oyster used what was within it to secrete a smooth, hard crystalline substance around what had entered its shell to irritate it. When we have challenges, we too are irritated but, like the oyster, we too have a hard crystalline substance within us to encase the irritator. *"..but the Father that dwelleth in me, he doeth the works."* (John 14: 10, KJV)

The oyster, an intelligent creature, knows how to defend itself against unwanted particles by going inward and developing something beautiful. We too know how to defend ourselves against challenges by going inward to develop something beautiful, but sometimes we forget.

At the end of any challenge, we will not be the same persons as we were. We will be transformed. We will be changed. If our challenge, like cancer, is life-threatening, we tend to review our life and vow to live it better. This clears the way for greater good. This transformation takes place on the inside and is a new course of direction or an opportunity for improvement. When things are going right we see no need to ask "why", because we are in a stagnant state of life. Life, like a river, is to keep flowing.

Life continually challenges us to greater growth, to greater expansion of ourselves, because it wants us to know who and what we are - love. As we face our challenges, take comfort from this: *"For I know the thoughts that I think toward you, saith the Lord, thoughts of peace, and not of evil, to give you an expected end"* (Jeremiah 29: 11, KJV).

Giving thanks says that you appreciate and are grateful for all that has happened to you during your challenge as transformation would have taken place. You are also grateful that as a result of this transformation, you are a greater person. We hold Thanksgiving Services to show our gratitude to our Creator when unexpected goodness takes place, like recovery from illness. The favorite songs are "How Great Thou Art" and "Awesome God". Yes. Our Creator is both great and awesome for it is through Him we receive our healing.

Do give thanks always for *all* things.

AFTERWORD

If any man defile the temple of God, him shall God
destroy; for the temple of God is holy, which temple ye are.
(1 Corinthians 3: 17, KJV)

It has always been my belief that nothing should be growing
inside the body. It should be as it was created with all its
systems in place, for my Creator designed my body to be in
perfect health.

I was involved in a motor car accident at twenty years of
age. When I visited the doctor, he asked certain questions
to which I was unable to give answers. It was so many years
ago that I do not remember any of the questions. He told me
that I should record things that happened to me. From then
onwards, I recorded the good and the bad on bits of pieces of
paper, keeping them in a drawer. I did the same thing with
my diagnosis of cancer, recording my experience, thoughts
and information on bits of pieces of paper.

I thought I should share the experience and information
collected with others who were experiencing the same thing.

When I mentioned to two friends my intention of writing a book on my experience with cancer from my bits of pieces of paper, they both asked for a copy.

After about a year of non-publication, I informed them of my intention not to publish because there were so many books about cancer on the market. I thought one less would make no difference. Nevertheless, I gave them a copy of the manuscript.

Three years later I received this email from one of them: *"Gloria, I have to share this with you. Remember I told you that my friend's Mum was diagnosed with breast cancer? Today was the surgery. Of course my friend was terrified. I remembered the article that you gave to me about how you handled your diagnosis. Could not find it. I wanted to read it. The day before the surgery I said I should share it with her. I said that you will not mind.*

Would you believe that I went looking for a book and there was the folder in a basket? I gave it to her to read and asked her to return it the next day which she did. She was blown away by it. Her comments were: "Very interesting. Gloria should publish this manual. Thanks for sharing."

This is how the book came into being.

BIBLIOGRAPHY

AHCC Research Association

Cancerbush.org.uk

Carper, Jean
    THE MIRACLE HEART. New York: Harper Collins Publishers Inc., 2000.

Carper, Jean
    YOUR MIRACLE BRAIN. New York: Harper Collins Publishers Inc., 2001.

Chopra, Deepak, M.D.
    QUANTUM HEALING. New York: Bantam Books, 1989.

Northrup, Christiane, M.D.
    WOMEN'S BODIES, WOMEN'S WISDOM. New York: Bantam Books, 1998.

Orloff, Judith, M.D.
    INTUITIVE HEALING. New York: Crown Business, 2000.

Pocket Anatomica
    BODY ATLAS. Vancouver: Raincoast Books, 2002

The Editors of Prevention
    HEALING WITH VITAMINS. Pennsylvania: Rodale Press, Inc., 1998.

The Tobago Writers Guild
    TOBAGO IN PRINT, Xlibris, 2015.